Differential Diagnosis in
NEUROLOGY

Differential Diagnosis in NEUROLOGY

Rajendra B Kenkre MD FRS
Neurologist, Goa
India

JAYPEE BROTHERS MEDICAL PUBLISHERS (P) LTD

Mumbai • St Louis (USA) • Panama City (Panama) • London (UK) • New Delhi • Chennai • Ahmedabad • Bengaluru • Hyderabad • Kochi • Kolkata • Lucknow • Nagpur

Published by

Jitendar P Vij

Jaypee Brothers Medical Publishers (P) Ltd

Corporate Office

4838/24 Ansari Road, Daryaganj, **New Delhi** - 110002, India, Phone: +91-11-43574357, Fax: +91-11-43574314

Registered Office

B-3 EMCA House, 23/23B Ansari Road, Daryaganj, **New Delhi** - 110 002, India
Phones: +91-11-23272143, +91-11-23272703, +91-11-23282021
+91-11-23245672, Rel: +91-11-32558559, Fax: +91-11-23276490, +91-11-23245683
e-mail: jaypee@jaypeebrothers.com, Website: www.jaypeebrothers.com

Offices in India

- **Ahmedabad**, Phone: Rel: +91-79-32988717, e-mail: ahmedabad@jaypeebrothers.com
- **Bengaluru**, Phone: Rel: +91-80-32714073, e-mail: bangalore@jaypeebrothers.com
- **Chennai**, Phone: Rel: +91-44-32972089, e-mail: chennai@jaypeebrothers.com
- **Hyderabad**, Phone: Rel:+91-40-32940929, e-mail: hyderabad@jaypeebrothers.com
- **Kochi**, Phone: +91-484-2395740, e-mail: kochi@jaypeebrothers.com
- **Kolkata**, Phone: +91-33-22276415, e-mail: kolkata@jaypeebrothers.com
- **Lucknow**, Phone: +91-522-3040554, e-mail: lucknow@jaypeebrothers.com
- **Mumbai**, Phone: Rel: +91-22-32926896, e-mail: mumbai@jaypeebrothers.com
- **Nagpur**, Phone: Rel: +91-712-3245220, e-mail: nagpur@jaypeebrothers.com

Overseas Offices

- **North America Office, USA,** Ph: 001-636-6279734,
  e-mail: jaypee@jaypeebrothers.com, anjulav@jaypeebrothers.com
- **Central America Office, Panama City, Panama,** Ph: 001-507-317-0160,
  e-mail: cservice@jphmedical.com
  Website: www.jphmedical.com
- **Europe Office, UK,** Ph: +44 (0) 2031708910, e-mail: dholman@jpmedical.biz

Differential Diagnosis in NEUROLOGY

First Edition: **2010**

ISBN 978-81-8448-947-7

Typeset at JPBMP typesetting unit

Printed at Rajkamal Electric Press, Plot No. 2, Phase-IV, Kundli, Haryana.

'A time to be born and a time to die'
For everything its season and
for every activity under heaven it is time

—Ecclesiastes

Preface

Neurology is a difficult subject in spite of advances in Diagnostics and Therapeutics since the end of 2nd World War.

Patients present with symptoms and signs which need careful evaluation to arrive at a Neurological Diagnosis. This book is author's approach to Neurological Diagnosis. The chapters are written and arranged in such a way as to give due weight to the subject under discussion in the 21st century, taking into consideration, Principles of General Medicine, Embryology, Anatomy, Physiology, Immunology, Biochemistry, Genetics and Neuroimaging: so as to increase the Diagnostic yield of a given neurological case under discussion and give impetus to clear thinking.

Drawings have been arranged in each chapter in such a way as to give Neuroanatomical and Neurophysiological meaning to the topics discussed on many diseases of the Nervous system which still need to be studied in greater depth in humans. The topics discussed in the text do not replace standard books and monographs on the subject of neurology.

I gratefully acknowledge the support and encouragement given to me by the publishers M/s Jaypee Brothers Medical Publishers (P) Ltd, New Delhi, India, in writing this book. My thanks go to Shri Jitendar P Vij, Chairman and Managing Director of Jaypee Brothers Medical Publishers, whose invaluable advice to me, to write this book has made me do extensive search of the Literature on the subject before structuring this book in a format that could be of aid to undergraduates and postgraduates in Neurology, bearing in mind that Neurology is one of the most dynamic medical specialties and there are more scientists involved in studying the Human brain than there are Physicists, Chemists, Astronomers and Environmental Scientists. It is also a fact to be reckoned with that as we look in the wider universe to find our place on the evolutionary scale of living life and receive and interpret cellular signals, albeit with help of aids such as artificial intelligence, computerized network of the Brain Model, it is the human brain with its millions of Neurons and its trillions of connections which does make the subtle difference in understanding ourselves from Immunobiological point of view, lest we take a wrong path in applying newer discoveries and inventions from the laboratory concerning human life.

Rajendra B Kenkre

Contents

1 Peripheral Neuropathy

DEVELOPMENT OF THE NERVOUS SYSTEM

The entire nervous system and the special sense organs originate from three sources each derived from *neural ectoderm*.

The first source is clearly delineated as neural plate which gives rise to central nervous system, the motor nerves and autonomic nerves.

The second source is the neural crest cells. These are migratory cells from the neural crest and contain mainly ependymal and mesenchymal elements and they form the entire peripheral nervous system including the somatic sensory nerves, the somatic and autonomic ganglia and adrenal and chromaffin cells.

The third source is the ectodermal placodes. This is a group of cells which originates at the edge of neural plate. They contribute to hypophysis, inner ear and the cranial sensory ganglia.

Peripheral Nervous System

Each spinal nerve is connected to the spinal cord by a ventral and dorsal root. The fibers of the ventral roots grow out from cell bodies in the anterior and lateral parts of the intermediate zone. Some enter the myotomes of the somites, some penetrate somites reaching adjacent somatopleurae, ultimately forming the α, β and γ-efferents. At level segments (T_1 - L_2) preganglionic sympathetic neuroblasm axons occupy these efferents at S_2 - S_4. Preganglionic parasympathetic neuroblasts accompany these efferents. The fibers of the dorsal roots extend from cell somata in dorsal root ganglia into the spinal cord and also extend into the periphery. There is continuous formation of neural crest cells along the luster of the spinal cord.

Blood Supply of the Peripheral Nerves

The blood vessels supplying a nerve end in a capillary plexus which pierces the perineurium. Its branches run parallel with the fibers connected by short transverse vessels. The peripheral nerves have two separate functionally independent vascular systems—an extrinsic system and an intrinsic system.

The intrinsic system runs longitudinally along the nerves and forms microvessels in the endoneurium. In the extrinsic system, there are neuritive and epineural vessels.

There is considerable degree of anastomosis between the two systems and this renders high degree of resistance to ischemia in the peripheral nerves.

Just as in the brain there is blood-brain barrier; there is a unique blood nerve barrier which is deficient in dorsal root and autonomic ganglia, and parts of the peripheral nerves. This barrier operates at the level of endoneurial capillary walls.

CLASSIFICATION OF PERIPHERAL NERVE FIBERS

Peripheral nerve fibers are grouped in bundles called fasciculi. The size, number and pattern of fasciculi vary in different nerves and at different levels along their paths. The structure of a single nerve cell is shown in Figure 1.1.

The classification of peripheral nerve fibers is based on various parameters such as conduction velocity, function and fiber diameter.

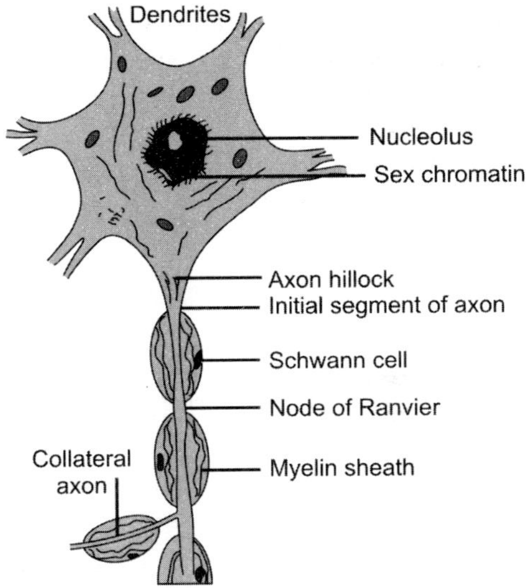

Fig. 1.1: Structure of a nerve cell (neuron)

The first classification system divides the fibers into three major classes designated A, B and C, corresponding to the peaks in the distribution of their conduction velocities. In the group A, fibers are divided into α (alpha), δ (delta) and γ (gamma) subgroups.

Group B are preganglionic autonomic efferents.

Group C fibers are unmyelinated nerve fibers.

Group Aα are largest and conduct most rapidly and C fibers are smallest and slowest.

Different types of changes that can occur in the nerve fibers including degeneration and regeneration are shown in Figures 1.2A to D.

Aα fibers (efferent axons) innervate cutaneous joints, muscle receptors and some large elementary enteroreceptors.

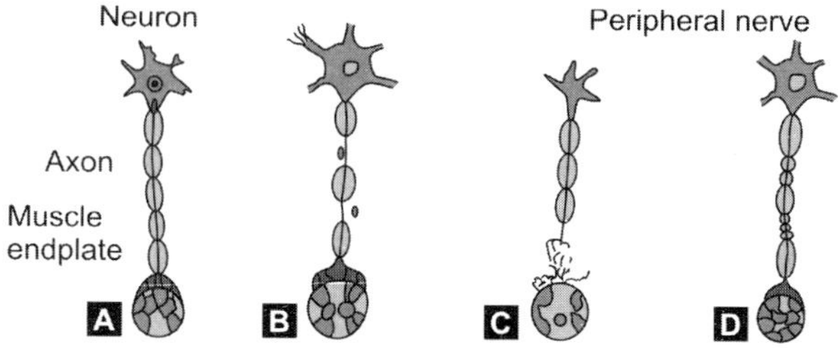

Figs 1.2A to D: Different types of changes that can occur in a nerve cell peripheral nerve: (A) Normal; (B) Segmental demyelination; (C) Axonal degeneration; (D) Regeneration after segmental demyelination

Aδ fibers innervate thermoreceptors and nociceptors including those in dental pulp. C fibers have thermoreceptive, nociceptive and interoceptive functions.

Aα fibers are up to 20 mm in diameter. They innervate extrafusal muscle fibers and conduct at the speed of 120 m/s.

Aγ fibers are exclusively fusiomotor to plate and trail endings on intrafusal muscle fibers.

C fibers are postganglionic sympathetic and parasympathetic axons.

Second classification system used for efferent fibers of somatic muscles divides myelinated fibers into Groups I, II and III.

Group I fibers are large (12-22 μm) and include primary sensory fibers of muscle spindles (Group I a) and smaller fibers of Golgi tendon organs (Group I b).

Group II fibers include terminals of muscle spindles with diameter of 6-12 μm.

Group III fibers are 1-6 μm in diameter have free sensory endings in the connective tissue sheaths around and within muscles and are believed to be nociceptive, relaying pressure, and pain in externally stimulated muscles.

Group IV fibers are unmyelinated with diameter below 1.5 mm. These include free endings in the muscles and are primarily nociceptive.

Nerve fibers (axons) are coated with short segment of myelin of variable length (250 to 1000 mm) each of which is enveloped by a Schwann cell and its membrane. The Schwann cell membrane surrounding the axon is myelin sheath. This axonal membrane has gaps called nodes of Ranvier which have specialized function containing high concentration of sodium channels (Figs 1.3A and B).

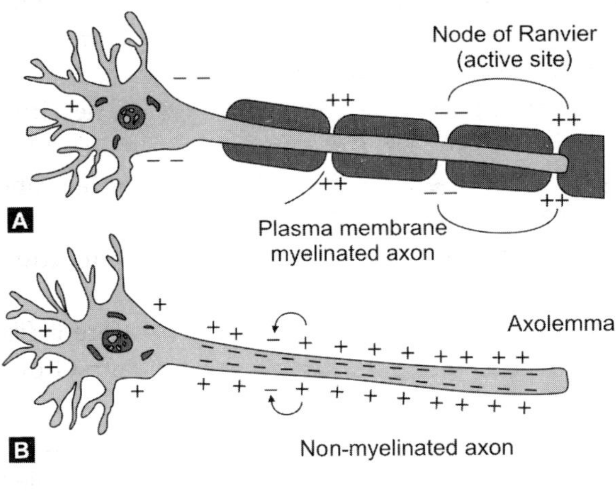

Figs 1.3A and B: Transmission of nerve impulses across myelinated and non-myelinated nerve fibers

GENERAL SYMPTOMATOLOGY OF PERIPHERAL NERVE DISEASE

Topographic and Clinical Patterns of Neuropathy

Impairment of Motor Function

This can be defined as persistent impairment of motor function over days, weeks or months which may signify segmental demyelination, axonal interruption, or destruction of motor neurons. Muscles of feet and legs are affected earlier and more severely than those of the hands and forearms.

Sensory Loss

In most polyneuropathies' there is impairment of both motor and sensory functions, but one may be affected more than the other. In Guillain-Barré syndrome, motor weakness is more pronounced than sensory loss although both may coexist.

In most sensory neuropathies, all sensory modalities like touch, pressure, pain, temperature, vibratory and joint position sense are impaired or lost. Vibratory sense is more affected than position and tactile sensation. It is even possible to delineate large fiber neuropathy based only on selective impairment of sensory modalities such as pain, temperature with sparing or lesser impairment of touch pressure, vibratory and position sense. This pattern resembles dissociated sensory loss of syringomyelia.

Small Fiber Neuropathies

Dissociation of sensation may extend over the arms trunk and even cranial surfaces. This pattern is typically manifested in neuropathies due to toxins, amyloidosis, congenital absence of pain, Riley-Day syndrome, and Tangier's disease.

Tendon Reflexes

Dimiuntion or absence of tendon reflexes is a sign of peripheral nerve disease. In small fiber neuropathies, tendon reflexes may be retained even with marked loss of perception of painful and thermal stimuli and loss of autonomic function. This is due to the fact that the afferent arc of the tendon reflexes utilizes the large heavily myelinated fibers that originate in muscle spindles.

Paresthesias, Pain and Dysthesias

This can be in form of "pins and needles", stabbing, tingling, pricking, and electrical sensation. In some sensory neuropathies, paresthesias and numbness are the only demonstrable features. There may be pain which may be of burning, aching, sharp, cutting, or crushing type. Sometimes, tactile stimuli may also elicit burning, tingling, or pain. Painful paresthesias and dysthesias are common in certain type of diabetic, alcoholic, nutritional and amyloid neuropathies.

Sensory Ataxia and Tremor

Ataxia may be pronounced when there is gross loss of joint and position sense as in diabetic neuropathy and variant of Guillain-Barré syndrome. Action tremor may also appear in certain phases of polyneuropathies, and large fiber neuropathies like those of immune mediated forms. Chronic inflammatory demyelinating polyneuropathy may give rise to coarse tremors.

Deformity and Trophic Changes

In chronic neuropathies, the feet, hands and spine may be deformed. This may be seen in hereditary sensory neuropathies. Important point includes finding of deformities like *pes cavus* or *talipes equinus* when the feet are pulled in that position. This is an important diagnostic pointer of neuromuscular disease of early childhood. Other changes may include trophic changes, diminution of hair growth in denervated areas, planter ulcers, etc.

Autonomic Changes

Autonomic changes include anhidrosis, orthostatic hypotension, small-to-medium sized unreactive pupils, lack of sweat, tears and saliva, sexual impotence, urinary retention and overflow incontinence, sinus arrhythmias and paralytic ileus. These changes correspond to degeneration of unmyelinated fibers in the peripheral nerves.

Fasciculation, Cramps, Spasms

Polyneuropathies usually do not give rise to fasciculations; they are usually manifestation of anterior horn cell disease. However, root compression gives rise to fasciculation, cramps and spasms and are frequently referred to as presenting manifestation with sensory neuropathies.

The differential diagnosis of peripheral neuropathies is better defined now as new epitopes on dorsal root ganglion cell, Schwann cell and peripheral myelin are identified and the corresponding genes are cloned. However, the diagnosis is still based on time honored criteria such as the pattern of motor and sensory loss, the time course, associated medical conditions, and exposure to toxins and drugs. Newer criteria increase diagnostic accuracy and effective therapeutic results. These are principally based on the fiber size involved in the peripheral nerve which is affected and on the genetics.

In small c fiber neuropathies, the predominant symptom may be burning pain and autonomic dysfunction. Group A delta myelinated fibers are also small sized. Symptoms, however, may be of different kind, expressed as lancinating pain, cold sensation, deep ache, there may be increased perception to pain and altered response to cold and heat. These small fiber neuropathies are associated with decreased sensation to pain and temperature threshold, minimal weakness and retained reflexes. Large fiber neuropathies, 12-22 m predominantly show motor deficit and impaired vibratory and propioceptive function. Thus, clinical presentation may be associated with impaired balance, positive Romberg's sign, loss of reflexes, ataxia of sensory type and proximal motor weakness. In general terms, both large and small fiber neuropathies have mixed features, which are motor, sensory and autonomic features.

SMALL FIBER NEUROPATHIES

Acute small fiber sensory and autonomic neuropathy.

Diabetes

In this type of sensory neuropathy small fibres 1 m, c fibers and unmyelinated sympathetic fibers are predominantly involved.

Clinical Presentation

Pain and temperature loss: This is greater than that of vibration and propioception. Reflexes are depressed to absent, there may be spontaneous lancinating pain, dysthesia, burning pain in the feet (c fiber), cramps of the feet and thigh, orthostatic hypotension, sexual dysfunction, anhydrosis, and small constricted pupils.

Mixed sensory motor neuropathy with some autonomic features: These form 70% of all diabetic neuropathies. In this form of neuropathy, small fiber modalities are involved earlier than the large fiber deficits. Hence, almost always presentation may focus on lancinating burning pain, or deep muscle ache which may later manifest with ataxia and features of diabetic pseudotabes, that is positive Romberg's sign, absent reflexes, arthropathy, foot ulcers, severe loss of joint position and vibration sense, and autonomic dysfunction manifested by decreased sweating, erectile dysfunction, nocturnal diarrhea and postural hypotension.

Diagnosis

Certain laboratory parameters are helpful in this form of neuropathy.

EMG: EMG may show early active denervation axonal features.

Laboratory investigation: Certain laboratory parameters are helpful in this form of neuropathy including fasting blood glucose values of 110-125 mg/dl. Random venous blood glucose of 200 mg/dl is positive for diabetes. Type 1 and type 2 diabetes can present in either form of peripheral neuropathy.

Diabetic Amyotrophy

Diabetic amyotrophy affects older patients with type 2 diabetes more frequently than type 1 diabetes. It usually affects patients belonging to age group of 50-60 years, in whom blood glucose levels remain poorly controlled over prolonged periods of time.

As with acute diabetic polyneuropathy, weight loss and anorexia is common.

There may be acute thigh pain which may later progress to quadriceps and adductor weakness. There is usually history of acute weight loss and general ill health, weeks prior to the onset of pain, which may be so excruciating that it may require the use of narcotics. Due to the insidious onset and weight loss, malignancy may be suspected. The condition usually improves over 2 years; nevertheless, it may leave sequela of wasting of quadriceps. The distribution of pain and muscle weakness suggests it is L2, L3, L4 roots that are damaged and not the femoral nerve.

Diagnosis

EMG: Associated axonal neuropathy may be observed in 50% of patients. Fibrillation potentials may occur early in the illness.

Laboratory investigation: There may be elevated CSF protein (mean protein 90 mg/dl) probably due to root involvement.

Differential Diagnosis

One often has to differentiate this form of neuropathy from motor neuron disease and polymyositis because of their insidious onset with chronic inflammation, and also from demyelinating neuropathy and malignancy in the pelvic region with lumbosacral root involvement.

Mononeuritis Multiplex

In few diabetics, this may present as cranial nerve involvement or intercostal nerve infarction. It is a type of vasculitis, probably due to immune complex deposition. There may be gradual improvement over a period of 12 months.

Generally, it is of acute or subacute type and painful onset with preceding weight loss in the setting of long standing diabetes mellitus. Cranial nerves III, IV, and VI, are most commonly involved. There may be partial involvement of III nerve with sparing of pupils. VII nerve palsy (Bell's palsy) is common in diabetics. Cranial nerves IX, X and XI are rarely involved.

Intercostal Neuropathy

This is commonly observed in older patients, males more than females, both in type I and type II diabetics. There may be pain and dysesthesias of burning type; complete sensory loss which may be unilateral, and focal motor deficits of abdominal wall.

Differential Diagnosis

- Herpes zoster
- Carcinomatous involvement of the nerve root due to lung Ca.
- Central cord syndrome.

Diagnosis

EMG: There may be fibrillation potentials in the paravertebral muscles.

Compression Neuropathy in Diabetics

Compression neuropathy in diabetics could be of the following types:

- Median nerve at carpel tunnel
- Ulnar nerve at cubital tunnel

- Peroneal neuropathy at the fibular head
- Lateral femoral cutaneous nerve
- Meralgia paresthetica
- Tarsal tunnel syndrome
- Radial neuropathy at the spiral groove of the humerus.

NEUROPATHY DUE TO HEAVY METALS

The heavy metals are often stored in the bones and other organs, such that slow release from this compartment occurs into the circulation after the cessation of exposure, resulting in development of symptoms.

There are many heavy metals which can cause peripheral neuropathy. Of these, few are discussed in detail due to their common exposure in the environment.

Lead Exposure

Lead exposure occurs in the smelting industry, battery manufacturing, disposal auto production, paints, lead miners, plumbers and soldiers who are exposed at firing ranges or when lead bullets are retained in the body. Both organic and inorganic lead is toxic to the nervous system. Inorganic salt produces neuropathy in adults which may be absorbed through inhalation, skin contact or ingestion.

Clinical Features

The patients may present with lead colic, intermittent abdominal pain, microcytic anemia, stippling of RBCs, renal failure (nephropathy), and bluish discoloration of the gums. Commonly there may be progressive motor neuropathy with generalized weakness and fasciculations.

Diagnosis

EMG: There may be decreased motor and sensory NCVS; slight abnormality of sensory nerve action potential; and axonal demyelination as evidenced by fibrillation potential and reinnervation.

Laboratory investigation: These include the following:
- Blood levels of 40 ug-100 ml
- Neuropsychological testing may be helpful as evidenced by decreased attention span, poor visual spatial processing, and loss of short-term memory.

Differential Diagnosis

Acute infective polyneuropathy and predominant upper extremities involvement may raise the possibility of autoimmune neuropathies (GMI) and hypothyroidism.

Arsenic

Exposure to arsenic can occur as a result of exposure to copper and lead smelting contaminated well water, manufacture of integrated circuits, and microchips. The absorption is through the skin, GI tract or lungs.

Clinical Features

Typical clinical picture following an exposure to arsenic includes gastrointestinal symptoms followed few hours later by distal paresthesia and distal muscle weakness. Areas of transverse bands (Mee's lines) are seen in the nails. The classical neuropathy begins one week after exposure and is usually associated with aching and burning pain spreading proximally from fingers and toes, and mild type of glove and stocking sensory loss affecting all modalities.

In severe cases, there may be a requirement for ventilatory support, especially when reflexes are depressed and absent.

In acute massive exposure, the clinical picture may simulate acute infective demyelinating neuropathy (AIDN), especially, when present with rapid ascending motor weakness and respiratory paralysis. In chronic exposure, there may be keratotic lesions of feet and hands with sensory neuropathy. Hyperkeratosis is seen in palms and soles and may simulate keratosis of neurosyphilis (Tabes Dorsalis).

Diagnosis

EMG: Distal axonpathy with absent SNAPs (Sural nerve action potentials) and reduced MAPs (Muscle action potentials).

Laboratory investigations: These include the following:

- Arsenic levels, greater than 25 ug/24 hrs are toxic.
- CSF protein is raised, but less than 200 ug% with no pleocytosis.

Mercury

Mercury occurs in two forms:

1. Elemental
2. Metallic

Elementary mercury in thermometers and metallic mercury is volatile at room temperature. Organic mercury is used in disinfectants and latex paints. Inorganic mercury salts and elementary mercury are used in dental amalgams.

There have been reports of major mercury intoxications in Minamata Bay in Japan. Organic mercury enters the body through GI tract. Elemental mercury may be inhaled. Effects of mercury intoxication on the peripheral nervous system are on the ganglions of the nerves and thus the patients may become ataxic. The polyneuropathy is of subacute onset, less than few weeks and presents principally as diffuse motor peripheral neuropathy.

Organophosphates

Organophosphates are used in the following ways:

- Insecticides: As a result, agricultural exposure is the most common form.
- Petroleum additives
- Lubricants

Clinical Features

Exposure to organophosphates may cause generalized motor weakness of acute onset leading to respiratory paralysis. Cranial nerve involvement may simulate poliomyelitis with bulbar involvement and Guillain-Barré syndrome. The differentiation between the two lies in the sparing of distal muscles. The recovery usually starts 5 to 15 days after exposure. The subacute and chronic forms are mixed forms of sensory motor neuropathy, with an onset 3 to 4 weeks after exposure. Prominent manifestations include ataxia and foot drop. Proximal muscles are also affected and there may even be autonomic nervous system involvement.

Thallium

Thallium is usually present in insecticides and rodenticides. As a result exposure may be due to accidental causes, with intention of suicide or homicide or sometimes food and water may be contaminated. Absorption primarily occurs through GI tract or skin.

Clinical Features

Paresthesias occur distally within 24 to 48 hours. Limb pain is more severe in lower extremities, increasing from distal to proximal areas. Other features include sensory loss, distal muscle weakness and atrophy, and loss of tendon reflexes. Sensory loss is greater than muscle weakness and both large and small nerve fibers are affected.

Diagnosis

EMG: EMG shows mild slowing of motor conduction velocities and evidence of motor axonal degeneration.

Pathology: Axonal degeneration affecting larger fibers, more than smaller fibers and distally more than proximally is observed.

DRUG INDUCED NEUROPATHIES

Most drugs after prolonged use cause degeneration of axons of the nerves distally. Discontinuation of the drug may prevent further damage.

Pathologic changes may occur in the dorsal root ganglion, cell body (neuropathy), myelin (myelinopathy). There is differential affectation of various degrees. Hence c fibers, A-alpha, and autonomic fibers may be affected.

Antituberculous Drugs

Isoniazid

Features: The neuropathy caused by isoniazid shows following features:

- Burning sensory neuropathy
- Loss of vibration, pain and temperature sense greater than that of position sense
- Deep pain
- Calf pains and fasciculation
- EMG shows sensory motor neuropathy.

Ethambutol

Features: The neuropathy caused by ethambutol shows following features:

- Sensory motor polyneuropathy
- Optic neuropathy with loss of green color detection.

Ethionamide

Features: The neuropathy caused by ethionamide shows the following features:

- Distal paresthesias
- Neuropathy is reversible after withdrawal of the drugs.

Antibiotics and Antimicrobials

Chloramphenicol

Features: The neuropathy caused by chloramphenicol shows the following features:

- Calf pain and tenderness followed by decreased distal pain and touch.

- Loss of deep tendon reflexes, ankle and knee jerks.
- Optic neuropathy may occur concomitantly with neuropathy.

Dapsone

Dapsone is used for treating leprosy.

Features: The neuropathy caused by dapsone shows the following features:

- Neuropathy occurs after prolonged use.
- Proximal muscle weakness
- EMG shows slowed motor conduction velocity with denervation.

Metronidazole (Flagyl)

Metronidazole is commonly used in the treatment of amebiasis, and bacterial infections.

Features: The neuropathy caused by metronidazole shows following features:

- Distal symmetrical, predominantly sensory polyneuropathy.
- Pathological examination shows axonal degeneration of myelinated and unmyelinated fibers. There may be segmental demyelination.
- Clinical presentation includes burning paresthesias and decreased reflexes.
- EMG shows slow motor conduction velocity and decreased sural nerve action potential (SNAP).

Misonidazole is a cell sensitizer used for cancer radiotherapy. Its sensitizes hypoxic cells to deep X-ray therapy and gives rise to similar type of peripheral neuropathy as seen with metronidazole. The dose at which normally neuropathy occurs is 50 gm/cumulative.

Nitrofurantoin

Nitrofurantoin is commonly used for treating urinary tract infections, with total toxic dose being 20 gm.

Features: The neuropathy caused by nitrofurantoin shows the following features:
- Axonopathy with rapid onset
- It may cause numbness in the distal legs followed by distal weakness and profound sensory loss
- Rarely profound motor neuropathy may also be seen
- EMG shows decreased motor and sensory conduction velocities and distal innervation.

Thalidomide

Thalidomide is used in treatment of leprosy, treatment of multiple myeloma, and HIV infections. 100-200 mg of single dose may give rise to symptoms.

Features: The neuropathy caused by thalidomide shows the following features:
- Predominantly sensory neuropathy tingling and numbness in feet followed by hands
- Hyperalgesia to pinprick
- Vibration and light touch is less affected
- Pathological examination may show loss of large fibers.

Cardiovascular Drugs

Amiodarone

This is an antiarrhythmic drug.

Features: The neuropathy caused by amidarone shows the following features:

- There may be motor, and predominant large fiber sensory neuropathy
- Distal motor weakness with sensory affectation due to combination of motor and sensory neuropathy
- There is gait disturbance
- EMG shows demyelinating and axonal features. There may be presence of decreased SNAPs (Sural nerve action potentials)
- Pathological examination shows loss of myelinated fibers; lysosomal inclusion bodies in Schwann cell, muscle fibers and capillary endothelial cells.

Hydralazine

Features: The neuropathy caused by hydralazine shows the following features:

- Distal extremity numbness and paresthesias
- Axonal neuropathy.

Enalapril

Enalapril is an ACE inhibitor.

Features: The neuropathy caused by enalapril shows the following features:

- Reversible motor-sensory neuropathy
- EMG shows prolonged motor and sensory latencies and reduced conduction velocities.

Streptokinase

Streptokinase may cause bleeding into the nerves, resulting in median and ulnar neuropathy which may be permanent.

Lipid Lowering Drugs

Lovastatin

Features: The neuropathy caused by lovastatin shows the following features:
- Myopathy is commonly seen
- There may also be presentation of cranial and peripheral neuropathy, which is seen concomitantly.

Simvastatin

Features: The neuropathy caused by simvastatin shows the following features:
- Fasciculations with proximal and distal muscle weakness.
- EMG shows reduced SNAPs (sural nerve action potentials) and normal nerve conduction velocities to mild slowing
- Pathological examination shows axonal degeneration of both large and small fibers.

Antineoplastic Drugs

Paclitaxel (Taxol)

This drug is primarily used for breast cancer. Neuropathy is dose dependent and may occur at cumulative dose of 200-250 mg/M2.
Features: The neuropathy caused by paclitaxel shows the following features:
- Sensory neuropathy
- Paresthesias of hands and feet followed by numbness
- Motor involvement in 20% of patients.

Vincristine

Features: The neuropathy caused by vincristine shows the following features:

- Neuropathy is dose dependent.
- Glove and stocking distribution of sensory loss.
- Symmetric distal muscle weakness.
- Loss of knee and ankle jerks.
- EMG shows low amplitude SNAPs and MAPs (Sural nerve action potentials and muscle action potentials)
- Mild slowing of NCVs (Nerve conduction velocities)
- Denervation and reinnervation noted with secondary demyelination.

Antirheumatic Drugs

Gold

Features: The neuropathy caused by gold shows the following features:

- Subacute progressive sensory loss
- Hyperesthesiae in the legs
- All modalities of sensation loss
- Distal muscle weakness
- Ascending sensory motor paralysis resembling Guillain-Barré syndrome
- CSF proteins are elevated
- EMG includes moderate slowing of MNCVs (Motor nerve conduction velocities) and SNCV (Sensory nerve conduction velocity)
- Pathological examination shows axonal and segmental demyelination.

Indomethacin

Indomethacin blocks synthesis of inflammatory prostaglandins.

Features: The neuropathy caused by indomethacin shows the following features:
- Sensory motor neuropathy, and sensory ataxia.
- Paresthesias of upper and lower extremities.
- EMG shows decreased MNCVs and normal sensory latencies.

Other Drugs

Allopurinol

Allopurinol is used for treatment of Gout and secondary hyperuricemia.

Clinical presentation: The toxicity with allopurinol shows the following features:
- Delayed sensory motor polyneuropathy.
- Glove and stocking distribution of sensory loss.
- Absent reflexes.
- Improvement seen after discontinuation of the drug.

Pathology: Pathological features of allopurinol toxicity include the following:
- Axonal degeneration
- Segmental demyelination.

EMG: EMG shows the following:
- Mildly decreased NCVs
- Decreased SNAPs (Sural nerve action potentials) and MAPs (Muscle action potentials).

Cyclosporine A

Cyclosporine causes reversible neuropathy associated with myoclonus and leukoencephalopathy.

Interferon Alpha

This is an immunomodulating agent primarily used in cancer patients.

Features: The neuropathy caused by interferon alpha shows the following feature:
- Mild sensory motor neuropathy associated with encephalopathy and myoclonus.

Pyridoxine (B_6)

Toxic dose is 2-6 gm per day but neuropathy may also occur at small dose.

Clinical presentation: Clinical features of toxicity with pyridoxine include the following:
- Numb feet and unsteady gait.
- Clumsiness of hands
- Perioral numbness
- Glove and stocking sensory loss
- Large and small fibers affected
- Decreased or absent reflexes.

EMG : EMG shows the following features:
- Normal motor and NCVs (Nerve conduction velocities)
- Absent SNAPs (Sural nerve action potentials).

Pathology: On pathological examination the following features are seen:
- Loss of large and small axons

- Axonal neuropathy with secondary demyelination
- Normal CSF.

Chloroquine

Primarily an antimalarial drug, it is also used as an anti-inflammatory agent.

Clinical features: Clinical features of toxicity with chloroquine include the following:
- Motor neuropathy
- Weakness predominant feature
- Absent or reduced reflexes.

EMG : Fibrillation potentials, myotonic discharges, increased recruitment.

Pathology: Segmental demyelination and remyelination of peripheral nerves.

NEUROPATHY ASSOCIATED WITH ANTIPSYCHIATRIC AND ANTIEPILEPTIC DRUGS

Amitriptyline

Overdose may give a picture of ascending paralysis as seen in Guillain-Barré syndrome.

Lithium

Clinical Features

- Short duration exposure
- Paresthesias distally
- Mild distal muscle weakness
- Depressed or absent reflexes.

Diagnosis

EMG: Decreased muscle action potentials (CMAPs and SNAPs), slow motor and sensory NCVs.

Pathology: Axonal degeneration (Sural nerve biopsy).

Phenytoin

Clinical Features

- Long duration exposure can cause peripheral neuropathy
- Loss of vibration and light touch in the lower extremities.

Diagnosis

EMG : EMG shows the following features:
- Axonal sensory motor neuropathy
- Decreased SNAPs and MAPs
- Slow NCV.

Pathology: Axonal degeneration and segmental demyelination.

Acetazolamide

This drug is used in patients with raised intracranial pressure, migraine and also as an antiepileptic.

Clinical Presentation

Painful distal extremity paresthesias and distal sensory loss.

Antiretroviral Agents

Clinical Presentation

- Distal sensory neuropathy

- Intrinsic foot muscle weakness with onset 8 weeks after initiation of therapy.
- Decreased pinprick
- Loss of ankle jerk
- Approximately one-third of patients may show loss of vibration sense.

EMG: EMG shows the following features:
- Low sural nerve action potential SNAP
- Quantitative sensory testing to quantify muscle action potentials is the better technique to follow course of neuropathy.

Alcoholic Neuropathy

- Occurs in more than 40% of hospitalized alcoholics both sexes equally affected.
- Pathogenesis of alcoholic neuropathy is related to nutritional deficiency, or direct neurotoxic effect.

Clinical Presentation

Clinical features include the following:
- Subacute onset of paresthesias followed by severe burning feet.
- Painful calves, cramps and distal weakness.
- Sensory ataxia.
- *Areflexia:* Autonomic dysfunction such as postural hypotension, anhydrosis, raised temperature, tachycardia and diarrhea.

Diagnosis

EMG: Distal innervation, reduced or absent SNAPs, mild slowing of motor NCV, prolongation of distal sensory and motor latencies.

Laboratory finding of significance: Decreased RBC transketolase activity, MRI shows central pontine myelinolysis.

NUTRITIONAL ASSOCIATED NEUROPATHIES

B_1 (Thiamine) Deficiency

This occurs in conditions of starvation, alcoholism, malignancy and dialysis.

Clinical Presentation

- Features of symmetric sensory motor polyneuropathy which may involve over weeks or months
- The clinical picture is of symmetric sensory motor polyneuropathy
- The paresthesias are distal and there is symmetrical absence of reflexes associated Wernicke-Korsakoff syndrome
- Rarely, there may be vagus and recurrent laryngeal nerves palsies
- Optic nerve changes are related to central scotomata
- Pathological examination shows axonal degeneration
- Laboratory findings show decreased RBC transketolase activity.

B_{12} Deficiency

Most often due to autoimmune induced intrinsic factor deficiency, vegetarian diet, blind loop syndrome, severe steatorrhea due to infestation of fish tapeworm.

Clinical Presentation

Clinical presentation includes the following features:

- Active large fiber neuropathy
- Paresthesias and burning hands and feet
- Cranial nerve I and II dysfunction
- Myelopathy, posterior column dysfunction
- Reflexes intact in the face of distal atrophy
- Psychiatric manifestation
- Recovery worse for vibration sensibility
- Paresthesias may improve.

Diagnosis

Laboratory: Laboratory investigations show the following features:

- Large hypersegmented neutrophils
- Low platelets a microcytic anemia which may be severe
- Intrinsic factor and parietal cell antibodies may be noted.

EMG: EMG shows mild slowing of motor and sensory conduction velocities, reduced or absent SNAPs (Sural nerve action potentials) distal low extremity denervation.

Pathology: Segmental peripheral neuropathy, posterior lateral spinal cord demyelination.

Vitamin B_6 (Pyridoxine)

Vitamin B_6 deficiency could be associated with nutritional causes, or isoniazid and hydralazine therapy, which inhibit conversion of pyridoxal phosphate.

Clinical Presentation

- Distal burning paresthesias in feet and hands
- Neuropathy improves with vit B_6 replacement or discontinuance of INH.

EMG: Decreased SNAPs, rarely motor axons are affected, slowed sensory NCVs.

Pellagra (Niacin Deficiency)

Clinical Presentation

Clinical presentation is similar to thiamine deficiency and includes the following features:

- Dermatitis
- Hyperketosis of the face, neck dorsal limb surfaces
- Diarrhea
- Dementia and axonal neuropathy.

Vitamin E Deficiency

Vitamin E deficiency could be related to chronic lipid malabsorption state occurring in abetalipoproteinemia, cystic fibrosis, short bowel syndrome.

Clinical Presentation

- Loss of vibration and position sense
- Limb ataxia
- Absent ankle jerks
- Proximal muscle weakness.

Diagnosis

Laboratory: The following abnormalities may be observed on laboratory examination:

- Measurement of alpha tocopherol in the serum by high performance liquid chromatography.
- Slowed sensory NCVs
- Decreased SNAPs.

METABOLIC NEUROPATHIES

These metabolic neuropathies are either hereditary or acquired.

Amyloid Neuropathy

The peripheral nerves may be damaged in amyloidosis by direct deposition of amyloid around the nerve fibers, deposition of amyloid in the myelin sheath and of vasa vasorum of the nerves.

This is a small fiber type neuropathy with pain temperature and autonomic dysfunction as constant features.

Familial Amyloid Polyneuropathy

It usually occurs as clinical syndromes with ethnic origins. It is commonly observed in patients of Portuguese extraction and also seen in Swedish and Japanese population. The Polyneuropathy starts in the legs in around third decade and runs a course for 10 years. It is painful, progressive sensory motor neuropathy. In Swedish patients, vitreous involvement is common. Men are affected more than women.

There are two other varieties: One of which was first detected amongst the British families in Iowa (USA) and other in the Finnish patients in Finland. The patients from Iowa show generalized polyneuropathy, while Finnish patients show multiple cranial nerve lesions and corneal dystrophy.

Diagnosis

Laboratory features: Biopsy of sural nerve, rectum and gums detects amyloid.

EMG: EMG shows axonal polyneuropathy in long standing cases. There is denervation.

Genetic diagnosis: By radioimmune assay and enzyme linked immunoabsorbent assay.

Differential Diagnosis

The differential point is presence of vitreous abnormality-vitreous opacities are common in familial amyloid polyneuropathy particularly those of Swedish and German varieties. Another point to note is presence of cardiac and renal involvement in amyloid neuropathy which distinguishes it from other hereditary sensory neuropathies such as autonomic sensory neuropathy. In toxic neuropathies, cardiac involvement is not seen but may show optic nerve involvement in the form of demyelination.

Diabetic neuropathies again show optic disk involvement and nephropathy.

A point to note is that Charcot joints are also seen in amyloid neuropathy like in leprosy, syringomyelia, diabetes, syphilis, etc.

Nonfamilial Amyloid Polyneuropathy

- Seen in patients with systemic amyloidosis
- Also seen in patients with multiple myeloma
- The clinical features are similar to familial amyloid polyneuropathy.

Porphyria

Porphyrias could be of various types:
- Acute intermittent porphyria
- Variegata porphyria
- Hereditary coproporphyria
- Aminolevuelinic acid dehydrase deficiency

Abdominal pain is the classical feature of porphyria; gene of hereditary coproporphyria is on chromosome 3.

Clinical Presentation

- Neurological complications of all porphyrias are similar and most attacks are provoked by drugs that induce the hepatic microsomal cytochrome 450 system.
- Starvation, alcohol, stress and hormonal changes may precipitate attacks.
- Abdominal pain is the most common symptom of an acute attack accompanied by nausea, vomiting and constipation.
- Agitation, nightmares and psychosis are common.
- Seizures could be generalized tonic/clonic.
- Axonal motor neuropathy.
- Ascending GBS (Guillain-Barré syndrome) with preserved reflexes.
- Ophthalmoplegia and other cranial nerves may be involved.
- Autonomic dysfunction, trachycardia, hypotension, pupillary dilatation, and hyperhidrosis are common.

Diagnosis

Laboratory findings: Features observed on laboratory examination include the following:

- Slight anemia
- High cholesterol
- Elevation of porphobilinogen in serum and urine
- Direct estimation of erythrocyte urobilinogen-1 synthetase is the diagnostic test.

Pathology: Pathological examination shows axonal neuropathy with patchy demyelination.

Differential Diagnosis

- Heavy metal intoxications particularly lead causes abdominal pain
- Arsenic nausea and vomiting
- Acute Guillain-Barré syndrome may resemble porphyria.

Drugs Precipitating Attacks of Porphyria

- Alcohol
- Barbiturates
- Chlordiazepoxide
- Imipramine
- Levodopa
- Methyldopa
- Phenytoin
- Tolbutamide
- Sulphonamides

Attacks of porphyia should be treated with intravenous glucose—at the rate of 10-20 gm per hour and hematin 4 mg/kg body weight per 12 hours, which reverses the metabolic defect. Chlorpromazine is a good sedative.

Lipoprotein Disorders and Peripheral Neuropathy

This could be of the following types:

- Metachromatic leukodystrophy
- Adult onset
- Juvenile
- Late infantile (most common).

Clinical Features

- *Infantile:* Age of onset 1-2 years; normal early development
- Neuropathy, absent reflexes, hypotonia, ataxia, progressive dementia, spasticity, dysarthria, in terminal stages, there may be myoclonic jerks and optic atrophy.
- Juvenile form: Onset is between 3-20 years; usually first decade. There may be behavioral manifestations, and depressed and absent reflexes, which may progress insidiously.
- Demyelination of CNS and PNS
- Adult onset occurs in 3-4 decades of life
- Dementia
- Optic atrophy
- Psychiatric and behavioral manifestation.

Diagnosis

Pathology: Pathological features include the following:
- Presence of Zebra bodies, prismatic inclusions, segmental demyelination and remyelination.
- Metachromatic deposits within Schwann cell and macrophages.

EMG: Demyelinating polyneuropathy with slow motor nerve conduction velocities; sural nerve action potentials may be absent or reduced.

Krabbe's Disease

- Onset 3-6 months of age.
- Arrest of motor and intellectual development.
- Optic atrophy and deafness.
- Loss of reflexes at later stage after onset of neuropathy.
- Tonic seizures.

Genetics

AR gene chromosome 14 (deletion, mutation, point mutation) Deficiency of galactosylceramide B-galactosidase.

Adult onset variant:
- Demyelinating sensory motor neuropathy
- Dementia.

Diagnosis

MRI: Diffuse cerebral atrophy

Laboratory investigation: Assay of galactosyl ceramide B galactosidase activity in leucocytes or cultured fibroblasts.

EMG: Demyelinating sensory motor neuropathy; reduced motor NCVs.

Pathology: The pathological features include the following:
- Multinucleated globoid cells in the cerebral white matter.
- Segmental demyelination with reduced fiber density of demyelinated peripheral nerves.
- Prismatic and tubular inclusions seen in Schwann cell and endoneurial macrophages.

Adrenoleukodystrophy

Genetics of the disease shows X-linked recessive chromosome inheritance involving XQ28.

Clinical Features

- Onset in childhood (4-8 years of age) in males.
- Cognitive decline, blindness, adrenal insufficiency, sensory motor neuropathy, seizures.

Diagnosis

MRI: MRI shows the following features:
- Cortical atrophy
- T2- weighted images: increased signal intensity, in centrum semiovale of parieto-occipital lobes.

Pathology: Pathological examination shows the following features:
- Demyelination of sensory tracts.
- Lamella inclusions in brain macrophages, Schwann cell and the adrenal cortex.

Adrenomyeloneuropathy

The disease has onset in adolescence or adult life. It may be preceded by hypoadrenalism and hypogonadism. The neuropathy is sensory motor demyelinating in nature.

EMG: Axonal sensory motor neuropathy.

Pathology: Pathological examination may show the following findings:
- Loss of myelinated and unmyelinated axons.
- Onion bulb formation.
- Schwann cell inclusions.

Abetalipoproteinemia (Bassen-Kornzweig Disease)

Genetics

- Chromosome 4Q 22-24 AR.
- Gene encodes a microsomal triglyceride transfer protein.

Clinical Presentation

- Onset during first-twenty years of life may be at first decade of life.

- Reflexes depressed.
- Ataxia, dysarthria.

Andersen's Disease

Clinical features are similar to Bassen-Kornzweig disease. There is absence of chylomicrons in the plasma acanthocytes in the peripheral blood.

Cerebrotendinous Xanthomatosis

Genetics

Chromosome 2 is location of the gene, encoding the enzyme sterol 27-hydroxylase.

Clinical Features

- Onset in late childhood or adolescence.
- Tuberous cutaneous xanthomas on extensor surfaces and tendons; achilles tendon and elbows are often early site of xanthomas.
- Cataracts
- Dementia
- Ataxia
- Sensory motor neuropathy – axonal and demyelinating type, sensory > motor.
- Propioceptive loss
- Dysarthria
- Generalized muscle weakness
- Extensor plantars
- Sensory motor neuropathy with loss of temperature pain and touch.
- Pes cavus

- Scoliosis
- Cardiomyopathy in few patients.

Diagnosis

EMG: Slowed sensory NCVs.

Pathology: The pathological features include the following:
- Large myelinated fibers show demyelination
- Some axonal degeneration.
- Some lipid inclusions in Schwann cell.

Laboratory: The laboratory features include the following:
- Absence of plasma apolipoproteins B, very low density and low density lipoproteins are reduced.
- Reduced triglycerides and cholesterol.
- Acanthocytes in the peripheral blood.
- Deficiency of blood clotting factors (Vitamin K deficient factors).

NEUROPATHY DUE TO STORAGE DISORDERS

Niemann-Pick Disease (Sphingomyelin lipidosis)

Clinical Features

Type I
- Disease of infancy
- Cherry red macula, choroid seen is red
- Hepatosplenomegaly due to accumulation of sphingomyelin in liver and spleen
- Dementia
- Seizures
- Although neuropathy is rare it is predominantly motor with sensory involvement. Decreased motor NCVs
- Segmental demyelination and remyelination.

Type II

- Mutation in sphingomyelinase gene on chromosome II
- Onset in childhood
- Hepatosplenomegaly
- No neurological abnormality.

Type III and Type IV

Neuropathy is present in type IV (Novascotia variant), onset in childhood, dementia, ataxia, vertical gaze palsy and hepatosplenomagly.

Tangier Disease

Tangier disease shows an autosomal recessive inheritance.

Clinical Features

- Swollen yellow tonsils due to deposition of cholesterol may cause difficulty in swallowing and breathing.
- High density lipoproteins absent in the serum with low cholesterol level.
- Small fiber neuropathy affecting myelinated and unmyelinated fibers causing severe impairment of pain and temperature sensation.
- Slow progression of neuropathy with absent reflexes.

Refsum's Disease

Also known as hereditary ataxic neuropathy, this is a phytanic acid storage disease. This disease occurs due to the inability to breakdown phytanic acid which is present in dairy products, fish, oils and beef. It starts in late teens and the clinical presentation is of visual loss, retinitis pigmentosa, night blindness, deafness, ataxia and progressive peripheral neuropathy. Icthyosis may be an early feature. Later, cardiac involvement may occur. Treatment is with low phytanol diet which may help modify the disease.

Fabry's Disease

Clinical Features

- Fabry's disease shows X-linked recessive inheritance. There may be presence of telangiectatic rash on the lower trunk and upper legs.
- Myelinated and non-myelinated small fibers are affected.
- There may be severe burning type of pain which may occur in paroxysms.
- Loss of reflexes.

In general when one suspects inherited neuropathies; the large and small fibers are affected with dissociated sensory loss; sometimes mimicking syringomyelia or cord syndrome. This should be borne in mind and appropriate investigations planned to arrive at the correct diagnosis of peripheral nerve diseases.

NEUROPATHIES DUE TO DEFECTIVE DNA REPAIR

Xeroderma Pigmentosa
Genetics: Chromosome 8 Genes

Clinical Presentation

- Onset between 1-2 years
- Increased sensitivity to sunlight

- Mental retardation
- Spasticity
- Deafness
- Dystonia
- Decreased lifespan due to associated malignancies.

Diagnosis

Pathology: The pathological examination shows the following features:

- Loss of myelinated and unmyelinated axons, with sensory fibers greater than motor.

EMG: Decreased SNAP (sural nerve action potentials).

Ataxia Telangiectasias

*Genetic*s gene localized on chromosome 11Q 22-23; unstable chromosome gene which spans 150 kilo bases.

Clinical Presentation

- Onset in childhood
- Telangiectasias on flexor creases by age 7
- Cerebellar ataxia, Basal ganglia dysfunction
- Distal motor weakness—propioceptive sensory loss
- Absent deep tendon reflexes
- Low IGA, IGE levels
- Glucose intolerance
- Impaired cellular and humoral immunity and increased incidence of leukemia and lymphoma.
- EMG shows reduced SNAPs with slight decrease of motor NCV.

Cockayne Syndrome

Genetics: There can be three forms of disease: A, B, C
- A: Chromosome 5 and XP
- B: Chromosome 10Q 11 -21
- C: Combination

  There are deficient repairs of the transcribed genes.

Clinical Presentation

- Photosensitivity
- Hydrocephalus
- Deafness
- Retinopathy
- Demyelinating polyneuropathy
- Hyporeflexia.

Diagnosis

EMG: Reduced motor neuro conduction velocity.

Pathology: Demyelination in PNS and CNS.

Laboratory investigations: Delayed recovery of DNA and RNA synthesis after UV radiation.

IMMUNE MEDIATED NEUROPATHIES

Guillain-Barré Syndrome

Acute inflammatory polyneuropathy.

Clinical Presentation

- Symmetrical leg weakness proximal greater than distal.
- Distal weakness develops after proximal weakness.

- Foot drop is rare.
- Onset to the time of maximal motor deficit is usually 3 weeks; it may be 50% after 1st week; 80% by the second week and plateaus to 90 to 100% by 3rd week.

Sensory Symptoms

- Early distal numbness and parasthesias.
- Severe muscle and back pain is seen 80% time.
- There may be cranial nerve involvement.
- Lower motor facial weakness is present in 70% patients and is usually bilateral.
- 20% patients have complete ophthalmoparesis.
- Oropharyngeal paralysis is present in nearly 50% patients.
- By 2nd week, 50% may have respiratory paralysis.
- In about 2% of patients there is urinary retention and 1% of patients have fecal incontinence.

Autonomic dysfunction: Autonomic dysfunction is common and may manifest as bradycardia, sinus arrest, supraventricular arrhythmias, hypotension which may be paroxysmal, paralytic ileus and areflexia.

Unusual Features

Unusual features include the following:
- Bilateral papilledema
- Increased CSF protein
- Severe ataxia where large peripheral nerve fibers are affected giving rise to ataxic tremor and loss of position sense.

GBS may be associated with transverse myelitis where there may be urinary and bowel involvement and asymmetrical reflex changes. Reflexes may be brisk in the upper limbs and sluggish to absent in the lower limbs.

Antecedent illness preceding GBS

- 2/3 patients have some history of antecedent illness, usually one week to ten days; rarely 5 to 6 weeks.
- Commonly, there may be respiratory illness, less commonly hepatitis, cytomegalovirus, Epstein B virus infection with headache, pharyngitis, pneunomia, dry cough or fever. Rarely, it may occur following small pox, rabies, polio vaccination.

Medical complications: Medical complications associated with GBS include the following:

- Cardiac arrythmias in 20 to 80% patients.
- There may be tachycardia, sinus bradycardia, ventricular and atrial arrhythmias.
- ECG may show depressed ST segments, inverted T waves, varying R-R intervals.
- Low sodium, (hyponatremia)
- Pseudotumor cerebri.

Early course: Prolonged distal motor latencies, conduction block with more than 20% progressive reduction in muscle action potentials (CMAP). Slowing of motor nerve conduction occurs as re-myelination occurs. Conduction velocities become slower. Slowed sensory nerve conduction velocities by 3 weeks of illness are associated with decreased sensory amplitude.

Sural nerve action potentials are normal but median and ulnar nerve sensory potentials are reduced or absent. Fibrillations may occur in about 20 to 60% cases in the first-four weeks. Abnormal spontaneous activity may be noted within 2 to 4 months in affected muscles.

In axonal form of Guillain-Barré syndrome, poor recovery is an important feature. Paralysis is rapid, CSF proteins are raised; sensory loss occurs distally, there is axonal degeneration and demyelination of motor nerves is absent.

Diagnosis

EMG: Reduced or absent motor and sensory potentials, nerves are inexcitable.

CSF abnormalities of note

- In general, up to 20 lymphocytes, if more cells are seen, one must bear in mind the possibility of underlying lymphoma, carcinomatosis.
- CSF proteins maximum may be up to 500 mg/dl usual levels are 100 to 180 mg/dl.

Differential diagnosis of GBS

Acute inflammatory myopathy: Painful muscles, diaphragmatic weakness, rare preserved reflexes and no bladder or bowel dysfunction.

Metabolic muscle disease: Periodic paralysis, no facial weakness, absent reflexes.

Myasthenia gravis: Affects facial muscle more than muscles of mastication; no sensory impairment; normal pupils.

High cervical cord lesion: These lesions cause flaccid quadriparesis. There may be loss of temperature control, loss of bladder and bowel control.

Variant of GBS: Miller Fisher Type

This may be present in 5% patients of GBS.

Clinical features: Clinical features include the following:
- Diplopia
- VI nerve weakness followed by IV and III nerve (Total ophthalmoplegia).
- Ptosis
- Ataxia
- Loss of reflexes
- Action tremor.

Diagnosis

EMG: EMG may show absent sensory nerve action potentials.

Laboratory: The following laboratory abnormalities may be observed:
- Increased antibodies to GQ1b epitope III< IV, VI (nerves); paranoidal regions are enriched with these epitopes
- CSF may show elevated protein levels.

Chronic Inflammatory Demyelinating Polyneuropathy (CIDP)

Clinical Presentation

- Onset and relapse are often triggered by infections.
- Onset commonly occurs in lower extremities; proximal weakness > distal; legs > arms.
- Touch and vibration sensibility are most commonly affected. Some have severe ataxia, propioceptive loss, and decreased or absent reflexes.

Diagnosis

EMG: EMG shows the following features:
- Motor NCV is decreased in two or more motor nerves.

- Absent F waves or prolonged F wave latencies in two or more motor nerves.
- Absent H reflexes and reduction in sensory NCV.

Laboratory investigations: The following abnormalities are observed on laboratory investigations:
- CSF increased protein 130 to 145 mg/dl.
- MRI shows enhancement of involved nerve roots and also of the demyelinating lesions in the brain.

Pathology: Sural nerve biopsy shows the following features:
- Demyelination in 80%; 20% are axonal and 15 % show mixed pattern.
- VER abnormality is detected in 50% of patients.
- CIDP is immune mediated disorder emerging from a synergestic interaction of cell mediated and humoral immune responses directed against incompletely characterized peripheral nerve antigens.
- An association with melanoma is of interest since both melanoma and Schwann cells derive from neural crest tissues and share similar antigens.

NEUROPATHIES ASSOCIATED WITH GENERAL MEDICAL CONDITIONS

Hypothyroidism

Clinical Features

Concurrent hypothyroid myopathy, pseudohypotrophy, axonal neuropathy, decreased mentation, trigeminal neuropathy (Pain), cerebellar ataxia, VIIth nerve dysfunction, distal sensory loss, burning and lancinating distal pain, muscle cramps, decreased relaxation phase of ankle jerk, hoarseness.

Diagnosis

EMG: Axonal demyelinating, decreased sensory NCVs:

Pathology

Sural nerve biopsy shows large more than small fiber loss of myelinated fibers, glycogen deposition in Schwann cells, myelinated and unmyelinated axons, endothelial and perineural cells, axonal degeneration.

Acromegaly

Clinical Features

- 35 to 45% have a peripheral neuropathy.
- Patients may present with paresthesias of the hands and feet.
- Legs are more affected than hands.
- Decreased light touch, vibration sense and joint sense loss.
- Reflexes are absent; concomitantly there may be type II fiber atrophy.

Diagnosis

EMG: EMG shows the following features:
- Decreased amplitude of sensory and mixed nerve action potentials.
- Mixed axonal and demyelinating symmetric polyneuropathy.

Laboratory: Laboratory investigation may show the following abnormalities:
- Raised insulin like growth factor, somatostatin – C and growth hormone.
- CSF normal.

Pathology: On pathological examination the following features are seen:

- Increased connective tissue in the perineurium and endoneurium,
- Decreased myelinated and unmyelinated axons onion bulb formation.

Hyperthyroid Neuropathy

Clinical Features

Proximal and distal leg weakness
Hypotonia
Areflexia in the legs.
Neuropathy is associated with propioceptive loss.

Diagnosis

EMG: EMG shows the following features:

- Slowed NCVs (both Motor/Sensory)
- Denervation of distal musculature.

Pathology: Pathological examination shows acute denervation.

Hypoglycemia

Clinical Presentation

- Motor neuropathy is distal and symmetrical.
- Upper limb more involved than lower.
- Wasting prominent.
- Dysthesia, painful paresthesias.
- There may not be sensory loss.
- Neuropathy is more frequent during hypoglycemic episodes.

Hepatic Disease

Clinical Features

- Peripheral neuropathy may be observed in more than 50% patients of hepatic disease depending upon duration of hepatic disease.
- Patient may presents with signs and symptoms referrrable to peripheral nervous system.
- Distal sensory loss involving the small fibers is more than large fibers.
- Loss of reflexes.
- The severity of neuropathy runs concurrently with duration and severity of hepatic disease.
- Autonomic features may form part of neuropathy.

Diagnosis

EMG: EMG shows the following features:
- Length dependent decrease of SNAPs and MAP (Sural nerve action potentials and muscle action potential).
- Normal NCV (Nerve conduction velocity).

Pathology

- Segmental demyelination, active demyelination or inflammatory cells are not seen.
- Myelinated fibers that are affected may reflect axonal degeneration and regeneration.

Viral Hepatitis

- Neuropathy is associated with both type A and type B hepatitis.

- GBS presentation may be observed in both A and B hepatitis.
- Mild sensory neuropathy.

Diagnosis

EMG: Slowing of NCVs during episodes of severe hepatitis B

Pathology: Segmental demyelination.

Tropical Sprue

Tropical sprue results due to nutritional deficiency and bacterial contamination of the small bowel. Improvement in the symptoms occur with folic acid.

Clinical Presentation

- Fatigue bulky stool
- Weight loss
- Glossitis, stomatitis.

Sarcoidosis

Sarcoidosis primarily affects lungs – hilar lymphadenopathy, heart, joints, skin, ocular and reticuloendothelial systems.

Clinical Presentation

Besides CNS involvement affecting spinal cord and cranial nerves, neuropathy may occur as isolated manifestation or as part of generalized disease.

Mononeuritis Multiplex

Clinical Features

- Polyneuropathy – Symmetrical
- Rarley GBS

- Predominant distal sensory paresthesias
- Anemia and megaloblastosis.

Diagnosis

EMG : EMG shows the following features:
- Decreased motor nerve amplitudes.
- Absent sensory responses SNAPs (Sural nerve action potentials).
- Denervation of affected muscles.

Pathology: The following features may be observed on pathological examination:
- Localized granulomatous nerve infiltration.
- Granuloma within the endoneurium of peripheral nerves, roots and cranial nerves.
- Changes in the blood vessels – angiopathy is a concomitant feature of sarcoid neuropathy hyperkeratosis.

Adults Celiac Diseases (Gluten enteropathy)

Clinical features: The following clinical features may be observed:
- Intestinal mucosa affected.
- Villous atrophy.
- Infiltration of the laminae propia with plasma cell and lymphocytes in jejunum and ileum.
- Increased HLA –B8 and DW3.
- Antibodies to gliadine.
- Distal dying – back neuropathy- fluctuating type depending on gluten exposure.
- Neuropathy may be associated with myelopathy and cerebellar degeneration.

Diagnosis

EMG : Axonal feature.

Pathology: Axonal degeneration

CRITICAL ILLNESS POLYNEUROPATHY

Uremic Neuropathy

It occurs concomitantly with multiorgan failure in patients who have been in ICU for more than four weeks. Sepsis may be an added factor.

Clinical Features

- Profound motor weakness.
- Absent deep tendon reflexes.
- Mild sensory deficit, often concomitant encephalopathy.
- Residual weakness in distal muscles.
- Profound loss of position and vibration sense.
- Decreased or absent deep tendon reflexes.
- Autonomic dysfunction.
- There may also be peroneal compression neuropathy.

Diagnosis

Pathology: The pathological examination may show the following features:

- Axonal degeneration; essentially large fiber neuropathy.
- Some segmental demyelination and remyelination.

EMG

- Decreased motor and sensory NCVs.
- When the uremic changes are reversed then there may be rapid improvement in NCV.

- Prolonged F-wave latencies.
- Denervation and renervation noted by needle EMG in distal muscles.
- Small fiber loss of parasympathetic nerves is more than that of sympathetic chain.

Laboratory investigations

- CSF is usually normal
- Creatinine clearance may be taken as an indicator for correlating EMG markers such as NCV; less than 10 ml/min of creatinine clearance is associated with decreased NCV.

INFECTIVE NEUROPATHY OR NEUROPATHY ASSOCIATED WITH INFECTION

Leprosy

Leprosy can be considered as the commonest form of sensory motor neuropathy due to infection affecting over 10-20 million cases worldwide. Leprosy is caused by lepra bacillus which is a gram-positive intracellular bacillus. Lepra bacillus reproduces at 26-30°C, and shows predilection for nose, testes, and superficial nerves – ulnar, lateral popliteal nerve, greater auricular nerve.

Lepromatous Form

Lepromatous form of leprosy is associated with abnormal cell-mediated immunity and disseminates hematogenously. Tuberculoid form, on the other hand is associated with the presence of cell mediated immunity.

Clinical Presentation

- Lepromatous macules, papules or nodular skin lesions.
- Symmetric rash of the face, forearms, buttocks, and knees.
- Loss of pain and temperature in dorsum of feet, ears, leg and forearm.
- Perforating ulcers at pressure points.
- Hoarseness of voice may be due to involvement of recurrent laryngeal nerve.
- Thickened and enlarged nerves including greater auricular, supraclavicular, ulnar, and median nerves.
- Patchy sensory loss in the face and trunk.

Diagnosis

Pathology: On pathological examination the following features are seen:

- Schwann cells of myelinated nerves are infiltrated by infection.
- There may not be an inflammatory response.
- In advanced disease, hypertrophy of peripheral nerves and increased levels of IL-4 and IL-10 are found in lepromatous lesions.

Tuberculoid Form

Clinical Features

- Tuberculoid form is characterized by the presence of anesthetic skin plaques, which show central hypopigmentation with erythematous borders in extensor surfaces.
- Disruption of nerve architecture.
- Intense inflammatory granulomatous reaction.

Borderline Form

Clinical Features

- It is intermediate between lepromatous and tuberculoid anesthetic patch.
- Borderline form is characterized by presence of hypertrophic nerves.

Diagnosis

EMG: On EMG the following features are observed:
- Axonal degeneration and segmental demyelination in affected areas.
- Slow NCVs and evidence of denervation of affected muscles.

Skin Biopsy

- Granulomas in skin, with or without bacilli.
- Nasal smears may reveal bacilli by special staining techniques.

Diphtheria

This disease is characterized by weakness of nasopharynx, oropharynx and diaphragmatic weakness, which is usually observed 5-7 weeks after infection.

Clinical Features

- 20% of patients have neuropathy.
- Cranial neuropathy involving the cranial nerves IX and X.
- Demyelinating neuropathy.
- Sensory motor neuropathy that involves the extremities.

Diagnosis

EMG: Slow motor conduction velocity.

Laboratory investigation: Positive culture for C-diphtheria.

Herpes Zoster

This can be described as latent dorsal root ganglion or 5th nerve infection, which is reactivated with immune deficiency such as in HIV infected patient and in patients undergoing therapy for malignancy.

Clinical Presentation

- Radicular distribution of severe lancinating pain.
- Decreased threshold to primary modalities of cold and pinprick in the affected dermatomes.
- Motor weakness may accompany sensory symptoms.
- Central features which may occur with radiculopathy include transverse myelitis and stroke in the distribution of middle cerebral artery.

Diagnosis

Laboratory

- PCR for Varicella Zoster Virus DNA is positive.
- *CSF*: Rarely glucose is less than 40 mg%; increased protein in CSF

MRI: Meningoencephalitis, and VI nerve involvement with dural enhancement.

EMG: Segmental denervation of involved dermatomes.

Hepatitis B and Hepatitis C

Neuropathy with hepatitis B and C infections may occur in isolation or in association with HIV infection or drug abuse.

Clinical Features

- Polyneuropathy.
- Small fiber neuropathy.
- Cryoglobulins are thought to cause neuropathy.
- Sometimes isolated nerve paresis in the form of mononeuritis does occur.
- There may be concomitant encephalitis.

Human Immunodeficiency Virus-1 (HIV-1)

Clinical Features

- 30% of HIV patients have peripheral neuropathy from disease or treatment.
- Neuropathy occurs in the form of distal symmetric polyneuropathy.
- There may be large and small fiber neuropathies.
- Painful Glove and stocking neuropathy in legs more than arms.

Diagnosis

EMG: On EMG examination, following features are observed:
- Reduced or absent sural nerve actions potentials.
- MNCV mildly reduced compared to amplitude.
- Reduced ulnar and median nerve motor and sensory NCVs.
- Prolongation of F-wave and H-reflexes.

Laboratory investigations:

- CSF proteins are elevated irrespective of seropositivity or negativity.
- MRI shows enhancement of lumbosacral roots, lumbosacral plexitis.
- Cytomegalovirus antibodies have been demonstrated in some patients with mononeuritis.
- *Pathology*: Pathology of nerve (sural nerve biopsy) reveals the axonal pathology of both myelinated and unmyelinated fibers.

This form of neuropathy has to be considered under various settings including the following:

- Acute inflammatory demyelinating neuropathy, GBS
- Chronic inflammatory demyelinating neuropathy
- Hodgkin's lymphoma
- Diabetes
- Alcohol abuse.

It may present as polyneuropathy, radiculopathy or mononeuritis multiplex. Central nervous involvement as encephalitis and transverse myelitis form concomitant clinical picture in large majority of patients.

NEUROPATHY DUE TO TRAUMA AND COMPRESSION

Classification

Neuropraxia – Axons are intact, but fail to conduct action potentials due to focal demyelination. Axonotemesis – Transection of axons, but the nerve trunk is intact.

Neurotemesis—Transected nerve trunk.

Sunderland Classification of Peripheral Nerve Injury

- First degree
  - Disruption of myelin sheath with intact axons and second degree nerve injury.
- Second degree
  - Transection of axons with intact stroma.
- Third degree injury
  - Transection of axons and endoneural tubes perineurium is intact.
- Fourth degree
  - Transection of axons endoneurial tubes and the perineurium fascicular transection occurs.
- Fifth degree
  - Transection of nerve trunk.

Prognosis of nerve injury depends on the following factors:

- Degree of injury
- Damage to the nerve.
- Distance from the muscle that is innervated.
- Wallerian degeneration.

ENTRAPMENT NEUROPATHY AT UPPER LIMB

Suprascapular Nerve

General Features

- Suprascapsular nerve comprises of C5 – 6 nerve roots arising from the upper trunk of brachial plexus and passes through the suprascapular notch.
- An entrapment usually occurs at suprascapular notch due to repetitive movements.

- Causes of entrapment include: ganglion cysts, metastatic disease, faulty positioning during surgical procedures, weight lifting, baseball pitches, etc.

Clinical Presentation

- Shoulder pain, if the nerve is impinged at suprascapular notch.
- The pain may spread to the superior border of the scapula towards the shoulder.
- Supraspinatus and infraspinatus muscle weakness.
- Weakness of shoulder abduction and external rotation of the arms.
- Wasting of infraspinatus.

Diagnosis

EMG: EMG shows the following features:
- Needle EMG demonstrates denervation in infra and suprascapular muscles.
- NCV with stimulation at Erb's point and recording over corresponding muscle.

Differential Diagnosis

- Musculoskeletal pains around the shoulder bursitis.
- Pericapsular fibrosis.
- Rotatory cuff injury.
- C5, C6 radiculopathy.
- Depressed biceps and branchoradialis reflexes.
- Brachial neuritis.
- Abrupt onset of pain may be bilateral.
- Brachial plexus traction injury (Tinel's sign) throughout the arm supra and infraclavicular fossae.
- Sensory loss and weakness.

Axillary Nerve

General Features

- Originates from the posterior cord of the brachial plexus; derived primarily from C5, C6, C7 roots (Upper trunk posterior cord).
- Innervates teres minor and deltoid muscles.
- *Pathogenesis of injury*: Dislocation and fracture of the shoulder; fracture of the humerus; surgical positioning causing entrapment in the quadrangular space.
- *Clinical presentation*: Sensory loss over the lateral shoulder, weakness of shoulder abduction and external rotation.

Diagnosis

EMG: Denervation of the deltoid and teres minor.

Differential Diagnosis

Orthopedic shoulder conditions; Brachial plexus injury.

Musculocutaneous Nerve Injury

General Features

Lateral cord of the Brachial plexus innervates coracobrachial and biceps muscles. Posterior sensory branch may anastomose with median radial sensory nerve and anterior sensory branch may anastomose with median nerve.

Clinical Presentation

- Weakness of elbow flexion.
- Decreased or absent biceps jerks.

- Sensory loss in lateral forearm.
- Pathogenesis of the injury: Trauma of upper arms and shoulder; fracture of proximal humerus and positioning during surgery.

Diagnosis

EMG: EMG shows the following features:
- Denervation of biceps and brachioradialis.
- Sensory conduction abnormality of the lateral antebrachial nerve.

Differential Diagnosis

- Brachial plexus pathology, C5 – 6 radioculopathy.
- **Median nerve compression at proximal humerus or in the region of the shoulder**.
  - *Pathogenesis:* Most common causes are traumatic anterior dislocation of the shoulder, and aneurysm of brachial or axillary artery.
  - *Clinical presentation:* The person is unable to pronate the wrist, there occurs paralysis of pronater teres, pronator quadratus, weakness of wrist flexion and ulnar deviation, paralysis of thenar muscles, and impairment of sensation to those digits which are innervated by median nerve.
- **Median nerve compression at the elbow just above medial epicondyle of the humerus**
  - *Pathogenesis:* Most common causes are trauma, direct injury, tumor, hematoma, elbow dislocated supra-condylar fracture. Hereditary sensory neuropathy with sensitivity to pressure and entrapment of the nerve at this level is rare than at the wrist. The second point where the nerve may be damaged is the point where the nerve

passes between the two heads of the pronator teres. Where the nerve gives off its anterior interosseous branch.
- *Clinical presentation:* Pain in the forearm, local tenderness at and below the level of supracondyle prominence where the nerve traverses pronator teres. At these two levels, paresis may be a prominent feature.
- There may be cramps in the fingers.
- The chief diagnostic feature is the weakness of long flexors of the wrist and the fingers.
- Other important feature at the low levels is inability to form O with the thumb and the index fingers.

EMG: EMG shows the following features:
- Denervation of medial forearm and hand muscles.
- Slowing of median nerve at elbow.

Carpal Tunnel Syndrome

At the carpal tunnel, median nerve is vulnerable and damage at this level is the commonest peripheral nerve lesion encountered. It is the commonest complication of pregnancy.

Clinical Presentation

The striking feature is that pain in the hand is severe at night and may be absent during the day. The pain is classically restricted to thumb, index and middle fingers. The symptoms may be relieved by arms swinging. Often, the pain extends to the medial forearm and occasionally as high as shoulder. There are four major presentations:
- *Pure sensory syndrome:* This usually occurs in women. There is objective sensory loss in the median nerve distribution. Pain may be absent. There may not be any motor weakness.

Consequently even by EMG tests. The syndrome is seen in women involved in knitting, sewing, crocheting, etc. especially if there are arthritic changes.

- *Pure motor lesion:* This is usually seen in men who use tools such as carpenters, plumbers, mechanics, etc. There may not be any sensory symptom. Patients present only with weakness of thumb for doing skilled tasks or wasting (thinning) of thenar eminence.
- *Autonomic presentation:* Autonomic presentation with severe pain is a feature of carpal tunnel occurring in pregnancy. Pain at night is a classical feature. The pain occurs in two phases. The hand may feel cold, clammy, swollen and as the arm is swung the pain is relieved. Stinging and the burning sensation is the feature.
- *Classical carpal tunnel syndrome:* This includes elements of all the above mentioned syndromes.

Diagnosis

EMG: EMG shows the following features:

- Decrease in sensory conduction at the wrist.
- Prolonged distal motor latency.
- Reduction of the motor and sensory amplitudes.

Ulnar Nerve Lesion

General Features

- Second most common nerve entrapment of the upper arm.
- Ulnar nerve comprises of C8 T1 roots and lower trunk of brachial plexus; some fibers pass through the medial cord. In the proximal forearm, the nerve passes under the humeral –ulnar aponeurosis between the heads of the flexor carpal ulnaris, which make up the cubital tunnel.

Common pathogenetic mechanisms for ulnar nerve injury are:
1. Occupational trauma.
2. Bedridden patients due to incorrect positioning of the forearm at ulnar groove.

General features of ulnar neuropathy: Effect on the motor symptoms is greater than that of sensory loss; decreased hand dexterity and strength; positive Wartenberg sign: Little finger is abducted due to weakness of the 3rd palmar interossus muscle. Pain may radiate to the elbow, medial forearm and wrist.

Clinical Presentation

- Hyperesthesia in the ulnar nerve distribution.
- Weakness of hand, fifth digit.
- Wasting of intrinsic hand muscles.
- Decreased sensation of the ulnar aspect of the palm.
- Tactile loss is greater than pin prick loss: distal two phalanges of the fifth digit.

Common clinical presentation of compression of the ulnar nerve at the wrist could be in the following forms:
1. Pure motor: Weakness of deep palmaris brevis, 3rd, 4th lumbricals, interossei,
2. Pure sensory
3. Motor and sensory; pure motor branch of the deep palm involves hypothenar muscles.

Diagnosis

EMG: The EMG shows the following features:
- Slowing of motor NCV

- Denervation of all hand muscles except those of thenar eminence.
- Denervation of all ulnar innervated hand muscles.
- Proximal lesion (to the wrist): There is involvement of the superficial and deep branches of the ulnar nerves and decreased SNAP.

Radial Nerve Entrapment

General Features

- Radial nerve originates in the upper arm, axilla. It comprises of C5-T1 nerve roots and also obtains contribution from all trunks of the plexus. Upper arm motor (triceps) at the elbow (brachioradialis, extensor carpi radialis longus and brevis.
- Radial nerve injury in the axilla could be due to crutch injury, lymphoma or tumor extension.

Diagnosis

EMG: EMG shows the following features:

- Focal slowing of the radial nerve in the upper arm.
- Denervation of radial innervated muscles in the forearm.

Clinical Presentation

Wrist and finger drop.

Differential Diagnosis of Radial Neuropathy

- Majority of the patients present with a wrist drop.
- At C7 radiculopathy – weakness of most muscles that extend to the wrist and fingers.

- At spiral groove or axilla – triceps is spared.
- If C5-C6 nerve roots are injured, brachioradialis muscle is involved. Triceps would be affected in C7 root injury.

ENTRAPMENT NEUROPATHY OF LOWER EXTREMITY

Sciatic Nerve

Sciatic nerve originates from L4 – S2 roots and is formed after the merging of the superior and inferior gluteal nerves. Lateral division is the peroneal nerve and the medial division is the tibial nerve. The pyriformis muscle passes through the greater Sciatic notch to insert into the greater trochanter. In 70% of the patients, Sciatic nerve passes under the muscle. Rarely, it may pass through the muscle.

Common peroneal nerve and tibial nerve separate from the Sciatic nerve most often in the mid thigh or upper popliteal fossa.

Sciatic Injury at the Hip

Clinical Features

- **Foot drop:** Peroneal component is more affected than the tibial component, resulting in the weakness of hamstrings, gastrocnemius and posterior tibial muscles.
- The ankle jerk may be depressed or absent.
- Instability of the foot.
- Decreased sensation on the lateral side of foot.
- Spared area around the medial malleolus.

Pathogenesis

- Sciatic mononeuropathy is uncommon.
- Most diseases affect the L4–S2 nerve roots, including lumbar spondylosis spondylolisthesis, metastatic disease.
- Hip replacement surgery
- Hip fracture – Injury occurs during close reduction.
- Severe direct trauma due to gun shot or stab wounds.
- Hemorrhage within the gluteal compartment.
- Hemophilia
- Anticoagulants
- Ischemic nerve injury
- Inflammation of the vasovasorum
- In the pelvis, the sciatic nerve may be damaged by direct spread of neoplasms from the rectum or genitourinary tract.
- In the buttock, misplaced deep intramuscular injection is a common cause for injury.

Clinical Features

- There is weakness of plantar flexion and dorsiflexion of the foot.
- It causes severe pain over the leg and foot.

Peroneal Nerve Lesion

Pathogenesis

- Common site of peroneal nerve lesion is due to the compression of the nerve at the fibula head, where the nerve winds around, protected by the skin and fascia.
- Trauma due to direct hit on the fibula.

- Sitting for prolonged periods with the legs crossed.
- In endemic areas leprosy is the commonest cause.
- Diabetes, polyarteritis nodosa and collagen vascular disease should also be considered when in addition to peroneal nerve, one or more than one nerve is concomitantly affected. This is known as mononeuritis multiplex.
- Whatever the cause, the patient will develop a foot drop and if the lesion is complete there is inability for inversion eversion and dorsiflexion of the foot.
- In most cases of peroneal nerve damage there is little or no sensory loss.

Tibial Nerve Lesions

- Tibial nerve may be damaged at hip joint and at the knee by trauma.
- In the calf it lies deep to the muscle; it becomes superficial as it divides at the flexor retinaculum into the medial and lateral plantar nerves.

Tarsal Tunnel Syndrome

A rare syndrome – designated as tarsal tunnel syndrome is described in which both the medial and lateral plantar nerves are affected. The medial plantar nerve supplies only medial aspect of sole with little contribution to muscle. Lateral plantar nerve supplies lateral aspect of the sole and has major contribution to intrinsic muscles of foot. In this syndrome, pain occurs over the medial aspect of the foot and the sole. It is of burning quality and is experienced on tapping the nerve below the medial malleolus. This can be considered as a positive sign.

Meralgia Paresthetica

- Meralgia paresthetica occurs due to entraptment of lateral cutaneous nerve of the thigh.
- Paresthesia occur in the form of numbness, tingling, burning, and hypersensitivity over the middle lateral thigh.
- It is usually of idiopathic nature; nevertheless contributory cause may be profound loss of weight. It is sometimes also seen in late pregnancy. Local trauma can occur due to wearing of tight jeans. In majority of patients, the condition remits spontaneously.
- Surgical decompression may be considered to release the entraped nerve.

2 Radiculopathy

UPPER EXTREMITIES

It is essential to delineate as to whether the clinical picture is that of single nerve lesion or root lesion. Sensory symptoms may be unreliable markers, for instance root lesion may give rise to paresthesias like tingling numbness exactly similar to that of the peripheral nerve lesion.

Exception to the generality is the rule in the following situations root lesions:

- C5: Pain occurs over the shoulder and into the lateral arm; it does not extend below the elbow.
- C6: Deep aching pain in the biceps muscle spreads down to the lateral forearm, involving thumb and index finger on both palmar and dorsal aspects.
- C7: Deep aching pain in the triceps muscle radiating mainly into the middle, index and ring fingers.
- C8: Root pain: It occurs below the olecranon – radiating to the little and ring fingers.
- T1: Root pain, deep aching pain at the shoulder joint and axilla, radiating down the medial side of the arm up to the olecranon.

Differentiation of Sensory Symptoms Root/peripheral Nerves

Three main nerves which are considered include the following:

1. *Radial nerve:* Detectable sensory loss in radial nerve lesion is limited only to slight tingling over the dorsal aspect of the thumb and index finger.
2. *Median nerve:* In median nerve lesion at the wrist, the pain besides involving lateral palm, thumb, index, middle and ring fingers spreads to the forearm and occasionally to the shoulder.
3. *Ulnar nerve:* In practice, the pain and sensory disturbance besides involving skin crease at the wrist, front and back of the little finger and medial half of the ring finger also spreads to the ulnar border of the forearm and this may mimic C8 root lesion.

Evaluation of Motor Function in the Arm

The first-seven cervical nerves and their corresponding vertebral bodies are shown in Figure 2.1.

C5 root lesion: Weakening of shoulder abduction.

C6 root lesion: Weakness of elbow flexion due to weakness of biceps and brachioradialis.

C7 root lesion: Weakness of shoulder adduction and extension of elbow and weakness of wrist flexion. Radial nerve lesion, on the other hand does not affect shoulder adduction or wrist flexion.

C8 root lesion: This causes weakness of long extensors and flexors of the fingers and in some instances weakness of small muscles of the hands.

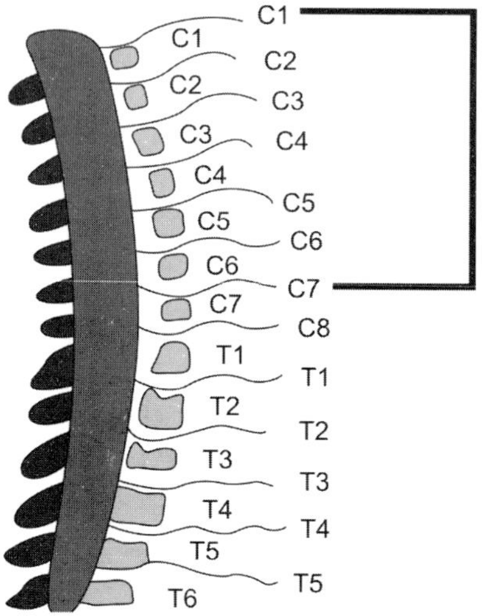

Fig. 2.1: The first-seven cervical nerves and their corresponding vertebral bodies

T1 root lesion: This causes weakness and wasting of all the intrinsic muscles of the hand. Among. 2-3% of patients, all hand muscles are supplied by ulnar nerve.

Clinical Syndrome

A few clinical syndromes associated with injury to the brachial plexus (Fig. 2.2) are described below:

Erb-Duchenne Type Paralysis

- It occurs due to the avulsion of C5-C6 roots.
- This can happen during forceps delivery or motor cycle accidents.
- It can result in the loss of adduction at the shoulder and loss of flexion at the elbow.

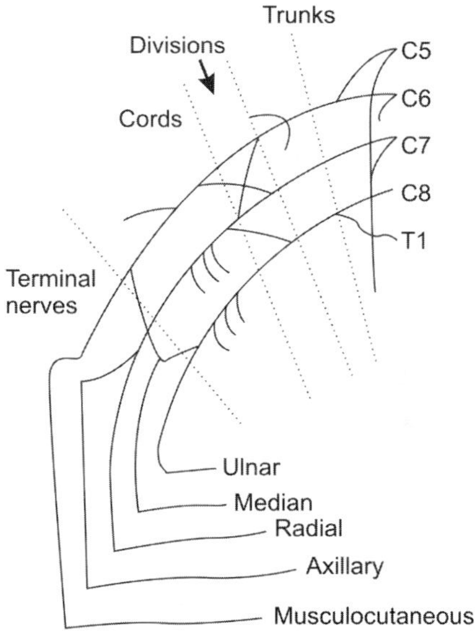

Fig. 2.2: Brachial plexus

Klumpke's Paralysis

It occurs due to avulsion of T1 and C8 roots usually, seen in injuries due to falls.

Root lesions due to cervical spondylosis
- C5, C6 roots are most affected.
- Biceps and supinator jerks depressed or absent some cases all three reflexes may be absent.

Acute Cervical Disk Lesion

- Severe root pain with radicular root pain.

Brachial Neuritis

- Typically excruciatingly severe pain over C5/C6/C7 dermatomes.
- Wasting and weakness of C5/C6/C7.
- There may be weakness of sternomastoid and trapezius.

Cervical Rib Syndrome

It occurs when accessory or the first rib is displaced upwards by distortion of the thorax, which could be associated with scoliosis, or thoracoplasty.

Sometimes could occur as an autosomal recessive disorder with malformation of the shoulder joint.

Symptoms

Neural

There is deep aching pain in the axilla and down the ulnar border of the arm, often extending into the hand, in the territory of C8-T1.

Principal affect is seen on abductor pollicis brevis. Nevertheless, it is important to note that pain mainly occurs in the ulnar deviated fingers and weakness and wasting is in the median innervated abductor pollicis brevis.

Vascular Syndrome

This occurs due to high cervical rib displacing axillary artery upwards.

There may be stenosis of the artery with poststenotic dilatation.

Clot may form in the poststenotic part of the artery and emboli may pass down to the brachial artery giving rise to ischemic changes akin to Raynaud's phenomena in the fingers.

Investigations

- EMG
  - Denervation of abductor pollicis brevis.
  - Normal median nerve action potential at the wrist.
- MRI
- Angiography.

NEUROPHYSIOLOGICAL AIDS

All neurologists should have detailed knowledge of electrophysiological techniques and their interpretation to assess a patient with peripheral nervous disease, which may be at the anterior horn, peripheral nerve or muscle. This would also help in providing sensible differential diagnosis in situations such as root lesion and peripheral nerve lesions. Certain terms need to be mentioned here for clarity.

Denervation: If the nerve supply to a muscle is damaged by disease of the ventral horn cell, nerve root or peripheral nerve, the muscle is denervated and EMG findings are denoted as **chronic partial denervation**.

Motor unit: Comprises of ventral horn cell, its axon and the group of muscle fibers.

Reinnervation

Sometimes, when a ventral horn cell or its neuron is damaged, certain muscle fibers cease to function and the surviving neurons branch out and take over the adjacent denervated muscle fiber activity. This is expressed in the EMG as **spontaneous electrical activity** as denervated muscle fibers are innervated.

On insertion of the needle in the muscle – insertional activity increases, that is injured potentials are prolonged and sometimes continue as burst of decreasing frequency, amplitude and pseudomyoclonic run.

Fibrillation Potentials

These are brief alterations in the amplitude of the action potential (50 - 200 μv). If prolonged and monophasic – positive sharp waves.

When the resting activity has been observed, the patient contracts the muscle gently, the inserted needle in the muscle is steadied, and individual motor units are studied.

Normal motor unit produces biphasic or triphasic potential up to 2 mv in proximal muscle and 5 mv in distal hand and foot muscles.

Giant unit polyphasic potentials vary from 5-10 mv up to 15 mv. The patient then contracts the muscle against resistance; the activity is continuous as the new units contract and rest. Obliteration of baseline sweep is called interference pattern. In a denervated pattern, gaps appear in the pattern. The surviving units are large and polyphasic, these are identical. This is known as reduction in the interference pattern and indicates denervation (chronic partial denervation), which may be due to involvement of anterior horn cell or peripheral nerves.

Nerve Conduction Studies

Muscle and nerve are the two things on which nerve conduction studies are based.

One stimulates the two end-points, one close to the muscle and the other at a higher point.

The time taken for the stimulus to travel from that nearest to muscle is known as distal latency, which in fact is time taken for the stimulus to travel from the nerve to end plate muscle and the delay which occurs at the end plate before contraction is elicited.

The nerve is then stimulated at higher point and conduction velocity is measured which is in meters per second and denotes the time taken by the impulse to travel down the length of the nerve.

Most peripheral nerves have standard velocity time commonly in the upper limbs, median and ulnar and in the lower limb, peroneal and tibial nerves.

At some points of injury to a peripheral nerve such as ulnar nerve at the elbow and peroneal nerve at the fibula, there may not be correct assessment of slowed conduction. In such a situation, we study action of quantitative muscle action potentials. Graded shocks are applied to the nerve at the wrist and ankle and muscle action potentials are measured, a few points below elbow and fibula and then above the elbow or popliteal fossa. It is the reduction from 10% at 1st mentioned points to 40% at the second mentioned points, which is diagnostic of damage to the nerve above the stimulus.

3 Disease of Muscle and the Muscle Endplate

MUSCLE DEVELOPMENT EMBRYOLOGY ANATOMICAL AND PHYSIOLOGICAL PRINCIPLES

Muscular system develops from the mesodermal germ layer and consists of skeletal muscle, smooth muscle and cardiac muscle. A motor unit comprising of alpha motor neuron and extrafusal muscle fibers is shown in Figure 3.1.

Skeletal muscle is derived from paraxial mesoderm which forms somites from the occipital to sacral region and somitomeres in the head.

Smooth muscle differentiates from splanchnic mesoderm surrounding the gut, its derivatives and from ectoderm (papillary muscles and mammary gland and sweat gland

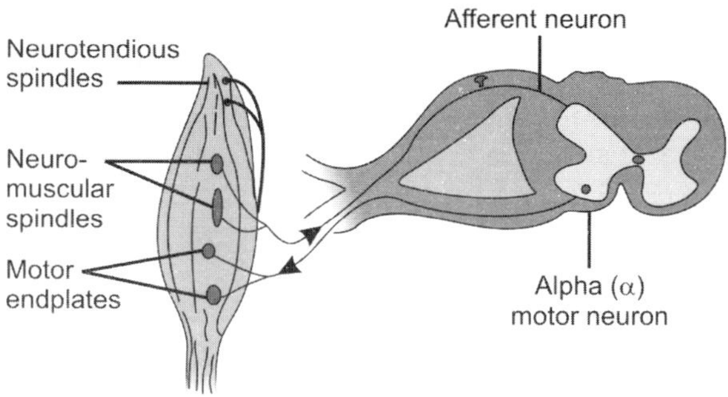

Fig. 3.1: A motor unit comprising of alpha motor neuron and extrafusal muscle fibers

muscles). Cardiac muscle is derived from splanchnic mesoderm surrounding the heart tube. Somites and somitomeres form the musculature of the axial skeleton. It expresses the muscle specific gene MYOD. The other region lies dorsomedially and forms the myotome. It expresses muscle specific gene MY5, myoblast, which form long muscle fibers. Recently, genes regulating muscle development have been identified. These include BMP4 and FGFS Wnt Proteins and the muscle specific gene MYOD. MYOD and MYf5 proteins activate the genes for mygenin and MRF-5 which in turn promotes the formation of myotube and myofibers. Muscle formation pattern is controlled by connective tissue into which the myoblasts migrate.

By 5th week of intrauterine life, cells which are likely to form muscles form epimere in dorsolateral part which reorganize as myotomes and the large ventral part the hypomera. The first indication of limb musculature is observed in the 7th week of development as a condensation of mesenchyme near the base of the limb buds. The myotubes express myosin iso forms, which are fiber specific. This myosin Type I increase significantly in first few years of life.

Muscles are exposed to varied changes in its normal formation expressed as inherited inflammatory and metabolic both (acquired, inherited) and toxic stages which results in clinical and subclinical presentation of muscle disease.

Differential diagnosis thus depends upon a careful family history and awareness of all diagnostic possibilities.

MUSCULAR DYSTROPHY

Hallmark feature of muscular dystrophy is inheritance factor which is observed to be affecting various muscle groups. The disease usually expresses itself as a period of quietness at various periods of human life. Recent evidence associated with electrophysiological and clinical studies points towards neurogenic component in the muscles disorders, which had been previously considered as primary muscle disorders. In majority of cases, clinical evidence suffices to make confident diagnosis of muscular dystrophy. Nevertheless electrophysiological, muscle biopsy and genetic studies are necessarily performed for prognostic purpose and counseling.

The following dystrophies will be considered in some detail:

- Duchenne's muscular dystrophy
- Becker's muscular dystrophy
- Fascioscapular Limb Girdle dystrophy
- Dystrophia myotonica
- Myotonia congenita (Thomsen's disease)
- Ocular dystrophy (Oculopharyngeal muscular dystrophy)

General Clinical Features of Muscular Dystrophy

- Family history: Only positive family history is of significance.
- Pattern of muscle weakness and the sequence, in which it is distributed, form the basis of classification of muscular dystrophy. Wasting in muscular dystrophy occurs at a later stage. Initially there is weakness and as the atrophied muscles degenerate, they are replaced by fat due to which the muscles begin to have a doughy feel and appear hypertrophied. In neural diseases, in which there is muscle affectation secondary to nerve or root or anterior horn cell disorders, the wasting is rapid and is usually seen concomitantly with weakness or may even precede weakness.

Reflexes are often depressed or absent very early in the course of muscular dystrophy, long before the muscle is significantly wasted. In terminal stages, clinical diagnosis may be impossible to make as widespread wasting weakness and loss of reflexes may well be due to neurogenic disorder.

Duchenne's Muscular Dystrophy

This disorder is usually seen in young males at the age of 3-10 years with the incidence of approximately 30 cases/1,00,000.

Clinical Presentation

Proximal muscles of the thigh, especially quadriceps and calf muscles are affected first, followed later by the shoulder girdle muscles. Neck flexors may also be affected at early stage and at later stage contractures develop. Ankle jerks may be preserved in early stage, whereas all other reflexes may be lost. Muscle strength of distal foot muscles inverters and evertors remain preserved. Facial and ocular muscles are not involved. Other features include macroglossia, and pseudohypertrophy of calves.

Investigations

- ECG shows tall R waves and deep Q waves.
- Ig levels may be low in 30% of the affected patients.
- Serum enzymes levels of CPK are raised.
- EMG is diagnostic.

Genetics

This disease shows X-linked recessive pattern of inheritance and is more commonly encountered in males. Rarely, female cases may also be seen. The genetic defect is seen in the short-arm of X P21 chromosome, which leads to **absence of muscle**

protein dystrophin. Dystrophin is normally involved in contractile function of muscles cells. Its deficiency destroys the mechanical stability of the muscle by affecting the sarcolemmal membrane, which results in rupture of the cell and influx of calcium.

Prognosis

The affected individuals are usually wheelchair bound by 12 years of age. Scoliosis develops early. Death usually occurs by 20 years of age, either due to cardiomyopathy, cardiac conduction defects or pulmonary complications. 25% of patients survive beyond 21 years. There is no curative treatment available to arrest the progression of the disease. Steroids have been observed to be of no proven benefit.

Becker's Muscular Dystrophy

Age of onset is between 5 to 15 years, rarely in the 3rd or 4th decades. Pattern of muscle involvement is same as that of Duchenne muscular dystrophy. Calf muscle pseudohypertophy occurs early; there is slow progression of the disease to the age of 30-40 years. Incidence of the disease is 1 in 30,000 male births. This disease also shows X-linked recessive pattern of inheritance. **However, there is difference in the mutation of X chromosome, which keeps some functional dystrophin active**. Other clinical features include:

- Right bundle branch block.
- T-wave changes.
- Fewer children have intellectual decline.
- EMG: Myopathic short duration small amplitude polyphasic potentials.
- Rare fibrillation potentials.

Cause of Death

- Respiratory insufficiency
- Cardiomyopathy.

Limb Girdle Dystrophy

This dystrophy shows the following features:

- Both sexes are equally affected
- Onset is between 10-30 years of age
- Proximal pelvic and shoulder girdle are mainly affected
- All proximal reflexes are absent.
- Ankle jerks are preserved.
- Differential diagnosis should include polymyositis and Kugelberg-Welander syndrome.
- Laboratory cardiac involvement is rare.
- Muscle enzymes are marginally elevated.
- Affected gene is on chromosome 4Q 35.
- EMG: Myopathic fibrillation potentials are rare.
- Muscle biopsy shows myopathic infantile forms demonstrating inflammatory changes. Molecular diagnosis is performed on DNA of leucocytes specifically.

Fascioscapular Humeral Dystrophy

- Most commonly autosomal dominant mode of inheritance; occasionally recessive
- Males and females are equally affected
- Usually affects individuals within age between 10-40 years.
- Incidence is between 3-10 cases per 100,000.

Clinical Presentation

- Weakness begins in the face then shoulder girdle, triceps, biceps and pectorals.
- Biceps and triceps reflexes are impaired.

- Slow progression.
- There may be minor disability.
- Deltoids may be enlarged as compensatory mechanism. It is true hypertrophy.
- Normal lifespan.
- Normal intelligence.
- Creatinine phosphokinase increased slightly in 50% of cases. Gene on chromosome 4Q 35.

Associated clinical features include the following:
- Ptosis
- Sensorineural hearing loss
- Cardiac involvement
- AV node abnormality
- Atrial flutter and fibrillation
- EMG: Myopathic
- Muscle biopsy: Myopathic
- Laboratory diagnosis: Molecular diagnosis performed on DNA of leucocytes is highly specific and sensitive.

Oculopharyngeal Muscular Dystrophy

This type of dystrophy shows worldwide distribution and mainly affects the chromosome 14Q 11-13. Both sexes are equally affected. There may be isolated ptosis with facial weakness and shoulder girdle weakness. 50% of the individuals have dysphagia. Associated features include retinitis pigmentosa in some families, visual difficulties, endocrine abnormalities, cerebellar involvement and cardiac involvement.

Laboratory: DNA testing is 90% specific and sensitive.

EMG: Facial, limb and pharyngeal muscles myopathic sensory and motor conduction velocities are normal.

ECG: Bundle branch block.

Differential Diagnosis

When ptosis, dysphagia and facial weakness are only features, particularly ptosis, myasthenia gravis is to be considered. In EMG, fluctuating weakness is the cardinal feature.

Kearns Sayre Syndrome

This syndrome is characterized by the presence of following features:
- Dysphagia
- Cardiac involvement, ptosis and ophthalmoplegia are predominant.

Myotonia Congenita (Thomsen's Disease)

Clinical Features

The clinical features of the disease include the following:
- Both sexes affected.
- Autosomal dominant mode of inheritance.
- Incidence is 2 cases per 100,000.
- Symptoms may be present since birth and include the following: Peculiar cry, difficulty in feeding, and inability to open eyes when the face is washed.
- Myotonia becomes apparent during second decade of life.
- Athletes may complain of slowness of grip stiffness. It is worse in the cold. There is usually muscle hypertrophy. Patients respond to drugs like quinidine, phenytoin, etc. Diagnostic clues are frontal baldness, loss of facial expression, ptosis and wasting of temporalis, masseter, and sternomastiods, which may occur early. There may be swan neck deformity, gynecomastia, gonadal atrophy and

impotence. Respiratory infections are common due to respiratory muscle weakness and abnormalities in immunoglobulins. Premature death is the rule.

Diagnosis

EMG: EMG shows the following features:
- Changes of myotonia
- Occasionally diffuse fibrillation potentials and fasciculations may be seen.
- Molecular basis of myotonia is increased muscle fiber expression of a calcium activated potassium channel and a possible alteration of chloride channel conductance.

ECG: ECG shows the following features:
- First degree heart block
- Atrial flutter
- Hypotension
- Sudden death
- Rarely, there may be posterior wall myocardial infarction.

MRI and CT may show non-specific abnormalities although ventricular dilatation and progressive atrophy are common.

CONGENITAL MYOPATHIES

Central Core Disease

- Abnormal structure and absence of muscle enzymes in the central areas of the muscle fibers.
- This disease shows autosomal dominant inheritance in which only type I fibers are affected.

Nemaline—Rod Myopathy

- Thread like structures are found in Type I muscle fibers.
- Usually shows autosomal dominant mode of inheritance; may also be recessive.

Clinical Features

- Fatal myopathy, weakness and flaccidity in infancy.
- Proximal muscles > Distal muscles.
- Facial muscles and muscles of mastication may be involved.
- Face may be elongated.
- There may be high arched narrow palate.

Differential Diagnosis

- HIV associated Nemaline myopathy: Pathological examination may show rods in myofibrils.
- Chloroquine myopathy; schizophrenia polymyositis; hypothyroidism.

Laboratory Features

- EMG: Myopathic
- CPK elevated
- Muscle biopsy: Rod bodies seen in atrophic fibers.
- Rod bodies may also be seen.

Myotubular Myopathy

Mode of inheritance is recessive sex-linked. Type I muscle fibers have a tubular structure similar to fetal muscle. Some patients may show autosomal recessive mode of inheritance.

Clinical Features

- Respiratory distress at birth, death, weak suck, weak cry, weak cough, weak swallowing and weak neck muscles at birth.
- Bilateral ptosis, and poor extraocular movements.
- Depressed or absent deep tendon reflexes.
- Cardiomyopathy.
- *Autosomal variant*: Limb girdle weakness which is usually evident by third decade.

Sporadic adult onset variant: Onset occurs in adulthood and is associated with slowly progressive weakness of both proximal and distal musculature.

Diagnosis

EMG: **Myopathic fibrillations and myotonic discharges may be common.**

Muscle biopsy*: Increase of perianeurysmal connective tissue. Small type I fibers normal type II fibers.*

PERIODIC PARALYSIS

Hyperkalemic Periodic Paralysis

General Features

- Genetic defect is on Chromosome 7Q 23.
- Mutations of the alpha subunit of the muscle voltage gated sodium channel gene.
- Complete penetrance in both genders is usual.
- Dysfunction or slow inactivation of sodium channels may be present.

Clinical Features

- Onset in 1st or 2nd decade (1-10 years).
- Generalized weakness (flaccid paralysis) which varies in frequency: Intermittent to daily which may last from 20 minutes to 1 hour.
- Attacks occur most often in the morning.
- These attacks are provoked by potassium, cold, fasting and exercise.
- Most commonly associated with myotonia.
- Potassium levels become 4.5-8 meq/L during the attacks.
- Areflexia.
- Myotonia may be seen concomitantly.
- Cranial nerves and respiratory muscles are spared.

Diagnosis

Laboratory findings: Laboratory findings are as follows:
- Calcium levels are depressed.
- ECG : Hyperkalemic changes.
- EMG: Myotonia, with high frequency discharges and occasional fibrillations.
- Muscle biopsy.
- Vacuolar myopathy.
- Tubular aggregates may be seen.
- DNA testing may be of diagnostic value.

Hypokalemic Periodic Paralysis

Genetics: Chromosome 1Q 31-32

Clinical Features

- Onset in teens 7-21 years age
- Attacks may occur everyday

- Or sometimes twice a year.
- Proximal > distal weakness
- Paresthesias are common rarely there is thirst, oliguria Examination
- Flaccid paralysis
- Absent deep tendon reflexes.

Diagnosis

Laboratory findings: Potassium < 2-3 meQ/liter may be associated with sinus arrhythmias and bradyarrhythmias.

EMG:EMG may be silent during the attack and there may be no response.

Muscle biopsy: Muscle biopsy may show dilatation of the sarcoplasmic reticulum. Type I and type II fibers are affected. Tubular aggregates may be seen in type II fibers.

Salient Features in Differential Diagnosis

- Hypokalemic attacks are precipitated by sleep, high carbohydrate and sodium meals and last for hours.
- Hyperkalemic attacks usually last less than an hour and are complicated by myotonia.
- Potassium relieves or prevents attacks of hypokalemic periodic paralysis.
- South East Asians have a high incidence of hypokalemic periodic paralysis.
- Myotonic discharges on EMG are seen only in hyperkalemic periodic paralysis.
- Potassium levels are high in hyperkalemic periodic paralysis and low during hypokalemic periodic paralysis.

- Onset of hyperkalemic periodic paralysis occurs in childhood, whereas that of hypokalemic periodic paralysis occurs during the adolescence.
- Andersen's syndrome is distinguished by presence of hypertelorism, short stature, broad base of the nose and cardiac arrhythmias.

Secondary causes of hyperkalemic periodic paralysis where on EMG myotonic discharges may be seen are:

- Renal failure
- Adrenal failure
- Metabolic acidosis
- Potassium sparing diuretics.

In these conditions potassium level > 6 meQ/L < 4 meQ/L and ECG changes closely follow the rise in potassium levels.

Thyrotoxic Periodic Paralysis

Genetics

- Highest incidence in patients of South East Asians ancestry.
- Older age (20-40 years of age)
- Provoked by high carbohydrate diet
- More prevalent in men than women
- Sodium channel inactivation secondary to sarcolemmal depolarization
- Loss of membrane excitability
- Improvement in restoration of thyroid function.

Disorders with Continuous Motor Unit Activity

- Myotonia
- Muscle stiffness
- Pain

- Contracture
- Cramps
- Fasciculations.

Origin

Spinal cord (stiff man syndrome)
Peripheral nerve (neuromyotonia)
Muscle (myotonias).

EMG

EMG shows the following features:
Series of muscle fiber active potentials
Positive sharp waves brief spikes continuous with motor unit activity – motor unit active potentials.
Decrementing high amplitude.

Malignant Hyperthermia

Genetics

- Chromosome 19Q 13.1 MH1
- MH2 chromosome 17Q 11.6-Q 24
- MH3 7Q 21 Q22
- MH4 3Q 13.1
- MH5 1Q 31 – Q32
- MH6 5P mutation.

Clinical Features

- Increased release of calcium causes severe prolonged muscle contraction.
- Occurs 1 in 50,000 adults undergoing anesthesia.
- Muscle spasm

- Generalized rigidity
- Rapid rise in temperature > 105° F
- Cardiac arrhythmias.

Inclusion Body Myositis

- Incidence is increasing
- Second most common form of inflammatory myopathy
- Commonly occurs over 50 years of age
- Male preponderance
- Duration of symptoms more than 7 years
- Swallowing abnormalities, and poor response to steroids.

METABOLIC MUSCLE DISEASE

Metabolic muscle disease presents as exercise intolerance, cramps and myoglobinuria with or after strenuous exercise or may present as progressive weakness. Type II muscle fibers are involved.

There are many metabolic muscle diseases:

- Disorders of glycogen metabolism
  - Acid maltase deficiency
  - Phosphofructokinase deficiency
  - Lactate dehydrogenase deficiency
  - Myophosphorylase deficiency (McArdle's disease).
- Disorders of lipid metabolism
  - Carnitine deficiency
  - Lipid storage myopathies
- Mitochondrial dysfunction with or without progressive weakness:
  - Luft's disease.
  - Kearns Sayre syndrome

- Progressive external ophthalmoplegia
- Phosphorylase deficiency
- Type V McArdle's disease.

Genetics

- Chromosome 11 mutations are common
- Stored glycogen accumulates at the sarcolemma areas of muscle fibers.

Clinical Presentation

- Exercise intolerance
- Muscle pain
- Early fatigue
- Sustained exercise precipitates symptoms relieved by rest.
- Any muscle or group of muscles including throat and masseters may be affected
- Myoglobinuria is common
- 25% of patients may have renal failure.

Diagnosis

Laboratory features: Creatinine kinase is increased.

EMG: EMG shows abnormally increased insertional activity, increased polyphasic potentials, increased myotonic discharges, and positive sharp waves.

ECG: ECG is nonspecific.

EEG: EEG shows the following features:
- Spike and slow waves in some patients who have seizures.
- Ischemic exercise tests of the forearm positive; no rise of lactate or pyruvate with exercise. In normal patients there is 3, 5 fold increase of pyruvate and lactate 1-3 minutes after exercise.

Pathology: Pathological examination shows sub sarcolemmal deposits of PAS postive glycogen and vacuoles.

Acid Maltase Deficiency of Childhood and Adulthood

Childhood

- Delay in motor milestones; proximal weakness > distal
- Respiratory muscles are affected early.
- *Laboratory feature:* Serum CK is increased.
- *EMG:* EMG shows myopathic features.
- *Pathological features:* Acid maltase in muscle is reduced; marked glycogen in muscle.

Adulthood

- *Genetics:* The most common genetic abnormality is mutations on chromosome 17.
- Slowly progressive myopathy
- Respiratory failure occurs
- Headache is common.
- *Laboratory feature:* Creatinine kinase may be normal or elevated.
- *EMG:* EMG shows the following features:
  - Myopathic
  - Increased muscle irritability
  - Fibrillations, positive sharp waves, myotonic discharges.
- *Urine*: Decreased acid maltase.
- *Blood*: Acid and neutral maltase activity in lymphocytes decreased.
- *Pathology*: Pathological examination shows vacuolar myopathy; all fibers are affected; acid maltase in muscles is decreased.

Lipid Storage Myopathy: Carnitine Deficiency (Secondary to Inborn Error of Metabolism)

In lipid storage myopathy abnormal amounts of lipid accumulates in muscle.

General Features

- Weakness, proximal greater than distal
- Eyelids, face and neck are involved in a fluctuating pattern.
- Heart and peripheral nerves are also affected.

Diagnosis

Laboratory features: Increased CK, serum carnitine levels are decreased.

EMG Myopathic

Pathology: Lipid accumulates in muscle, and liver, which is greater than that in heart and kidneys.

Associated clinical feature: Myopathic weakness may be associated with hepatic encephalopathy.

ABNORMAL GLYCOGEN METABOLISM

Pompe's Disease

Clinical Features

- Disease of infancy and usually fatal.
- Inheritance is autosomal recessive.
- Affected gene is located on long arm of chromosome 17.
- Cardiac damage is common
- Large tongue.

Diagnosis

Muscle biopsy: The following features are observed:

- Glycogen filled vacuoles occur throughout the muscle cells.
- Labile blood pressure
- *Laboratory features*: Elevated CPK>10,000 units
- Increased potassium levels
- Lactic acidosis.

INFLAMMATORY MYOPATHY

Three major forms are:

- Polymyositis
- Dermatomyositis
- Inclusion body myositis.

An example of similar pattern of affectation of muscle as inflammatory myopathies is collagen vascular disease. In these diseases, however, extraocular muscle involvement is common.

Polymyositis

Clinical Features

- Possible increased incidence of HLAB8 and B12 antigen
- Subacute onset occurring within weeks to months
- Younger age of onset 5-14 years, adult onset may be between 45-65 years
- Incidence 1:1,00,000 people
- Females > Males
- Neck flexors weakness
- Symmetrical proximal girdle weakness.
- Dysphagia occurs in 20-30% patients due to involvement of striated posterior pharyngeal and cricopharyngeous muscle

- Respiratory involvement is rare.
- Associations with many forms of malignancies and connective tissue disorders.
- Cardiac involvement does occur
  - *ECG:* Nonspecific ST-T wave abnormalities
  - *Heart block:* Bundle branch block
- Polymyositis may be associated with Systemic Lupus Erythematous
  - Muscle involvement shows same distribution as in polymyositis.
  - Cerebral arteritis, arthritis, and pericarditis may be present.
- Severe joint involvement
- Pattern of weakness similar to PM
- Associated neuropathy
- C1-C2 dislocation.

Diagnosis

Laboratory: The following features are observed on laboratory examination:

- IgG antibodies to double standard DNA are most specific
- CPK is elevated
- Rheumatoid arthritis antigens
- Type II muscle atrophy
- Immune complexes containing immunoglobulin and complement in blood vessel walls.
- Muscle enzymes are elevated by 5-50 times normal.
- *ESR*: Normal; or may be increased
- *EMG*: Membrane irritability; myopathic motor unit potentials.

- *Muscle biopsy*: Inflammatory cells in the perimysium and endomysium; single fiber necrosis; inflammatory aggregates contain higher percentage of T cells and small percentage of B cells; pathology is confined to skin, subcutaneous tissue and underlying muscles. Muscle biopsy may also show vasculitis of small blood vessels; Immunoglobulin deposits and complement found in muscles.

Dermatomyositis

Clinical Features

- Childhood variant involves individuals belonging to age 5-14 years
- Adults: Usually involved between 45-65 years of age.
- Onset occurs over weeks to months
- Rash may precede weakness
- Weakness is proximal symmetrical and involves neck flexors.
- Dysphagia occurs in 30% patients.
- Muscle tenderness < 50%
- Skin manifestation: Acute erythema and edema of subcutaneous tissues, which shows perioral, periorbital, malar, and chest distribution.
- Chronic scaling of the skin
- Hyper pigmentation
- Brisk to exaggerated reflexes in lower limbs

Systemic involvement shows the following features:

- Atrial arrhythmias
- AV conduction defects
- Bundle branch block
- Primary lung diseases

- Interstitial lung disease
- Secondary lung disease
- Weakness of respiratory muscles
- Chronic aspiration
- Dermatomyositis may be associated with malignancy
  - Very high association, almost 4 in 10 cases.
  - Patients are usually older than 40 years.
  - Malignancy may precede or follow myopathy usually by 2 years.
  - Small cell carcinoma lung in men and ovarian cancer in women are most common; incidence wise, stomach cancershows greater incidence than colorectal cancer.
  - Removal of tumor: Myopathy may regress
  - Recurrence of myopathy may herald recurrence of tumor.

Diagnosis

Laboratory features: The following laboratory features are observed:

- Creatinine kinase is elevated almost in all cases.
- Antinuclear helicase antibody is detected in 5-10% of patients.

EMG: EMG shows the following features:

- Myopathic
- Increased insertional activity
- Positive sharp waves fibrillations in paraspinal muscles.
- Long standing cases: Signs of reinnervation with high amplitude long duration muscle action potential.

Muscle biopsy: Muscle biopsy shows the following features:

- Perivascular inflammatory cells in the perimysium
- B cells and helper T cells in the infiltrate.

- Tubular aggregates are noted in the cytoplasm of endothelial cell of arterioles
- Capillaries show necrosis and degeneration.

Toxic Myopathy

Muscles may be damaged by direct toxic effects or secondarily from immune mechanism, electrolyte imbalance, and ischemia.

Major categories of toxic substances include the following:
- Alcohol
- Steroids
- Anti HIV compounds
- Vincristine and colchicine which have direct toxic effect on microtubules of muscles.
- Anesthetics.

Clinical Presentation

- Pain and myoglobinuria
- Generalized or focal weakness
- Wasting of affected muscle
- Cramps
- Cardiomyopathy.

Myopathy due to Nutritional Deficiency (Vitamin E Deficiency)

Clinical Features

- Cerebellar degeneration
- Posterior column loss
- Peripheral neuropathy: Large fiber type
- Proximal myopathy

- Vitamin D deficiency
- Proximal muscle weakness
- Legs are affected more than the arms
- Wasting pain and tenderness.

Diagnosis

Laboratory features:
- Increased alkaline phosphatase
- Normal CK
- Normal muscle biopsy.

Osteomalacic Myopathy

One-third of patients with osteomalacia have weakness or myalgia.

Causes

- Dietary deficiency or malabsorption of vitamin D
- Dilantin
- Renal tubular acidosis.

Clinical Presentation

- Insidious onset
- Proximal weakness
- Myalgia

Diagnosis

Laboratory features:
- Parathyroid levels are normal or increased
- Normal CK

- Decreased bone density
- Serum calcium phosphate and alkaline phosphatase increased.

EMG: EMG shows the following features:
- Myopathic in 80% of patients
- Slow NCV.

Pathology: Pathological examination shows the following features:
- Type II fiber atrophy
- Variation of fiber size
- Fatty infiltration
- Inflammatory macrophages and CD8+ cytotoxic infiltrates that are perimysial, endomysial and perivascular
- Nemaline rods may be found in muscle fibers.

Fungal Myositis

Fungal myositis occurs in immunocompromised patients due to; (1) *Candida,* (2) *Cryptococcus,* (3) *Aspergillus,* (4) *Actinomyces,* (5) *Histoplasma.*

Sarcoid and Tuberculous Myositis

Tuberculous myositis occurs in immunocompromised patients. Muscle biopsy shows granulomatous infiltration and presence of acid fast bacilli noted in the lesions.

Sarcoid myositis is associated with painful muscle weakness, proximal muscle cramps and neuropathy.

Diagnosis

Laboratory: Positive chest X-ray, with nearly 90% patients demonstrating hilar lymphadenopathy.

MRI of muscle: Distinctive star shaped pattern with peripheral gadolinium enhancement.

Cysticercosis

Causitive organism is *T. Solium*. The spread usually occurs via oral route, due to consumption of undercooked meat, pork, uncooked vegetables, etc. Mature larvae penetrate the intestinal mucosa and are disseminated by the lymphatics and hematogenously.

Clinical Presentation

- Seizures
- Meningoencephalitis
- Muslce involvement
- Weakness
- Pain
- Proptosis and ophthalmoparesis.

Diagnosis

CT imaging and MRI: Calcified cysts in brain and muscle cysticerci are identified.

Endocrine Myopathy

50-80% of patients with Cushing's disease develop muscle weakness and 3-20% of patients on steroid develop muscle weakness. Females develop myopathy more often than males. 30 mg of prednisone a day is required to induce myopathy.

Clinical Presentation

- Insidious onset
- Quadriceps and Iliopsoas are the first muscles to be affected.

- Proximal muscles are more affected than the distal muscles
- Facial and neck muscles are spared.

Diagnosis

Laboratory: CK is normal.

EMG: Normal insertional activity, low amplitude, short duration, polyphasic potentials muscles action potentials.

Pathological examination: On pathological examination following features are seen:
- Type II fiber muscles atrophy
- Electron microscopy
- Mitochondial aggregation swelling and vacuolation.

Myopathy of Addison's Disease

Muscle weakness is caused by decreased blood flow, impaired carbohydrate metabolism, and electrolyte abnormalities.

Clinical Presentation

- Primarily autoimmune disease; may also be caused by tuberculosis, pituitary failure and hemorrhage.
- Generalized muscle weakness, fatigue and cramps are seen in 25% of patients.

Diagnosis

Laboratory evaluation shows the following features:
- High serum potassium with loss of serum sodium
- Eosinophilia.
- ACTH stimulation test is positive
- EMG is normal.

Myopathy of Thyroid Disease

- Female preponderance 3:1
- Age of onset 50 years
- Proximal muscle weakness
- Weakness is out of proportion to wasting
- Muscle pain and fatigue are common
- Tendon reflexes are normal.

Associated myasthenia gravis may occur in 7.5% hyperthyroid, and hypothyroid 5%.

Diagnosis

Laboratory features:
- Decreased TSH; elevated levels of T3, T4
- CK, LDH, SGOT normal
- CK elevated.

EMG: EMG shows the following features:
- Short duration of muscle action potential
- Increased polyphasic potentials
- 30% of patients have abnormal EMG and have normal muscle strength.

Pathology: Pathological examination shows fatty infiltration between myofibrils, and atrophy of type I and type II fibers.

Hypothyroid Myopathy

General Features

- Decreased mitochondrial oxygen capacity.
- Reduced glucose up take and muscle enzyme activity.
- Fasting hypoglycemia, insulin resistance

- Glycogen accumulation occurs in muscles.
- Decreased adrenergic receptors on muscle cells which causes diminished glycogenolysis.

Clinical Presentation

- Proximal muscle weakness
- Muscle fatigue and stiffness
- Myalgia and stiffness
- Pseudohypertrophy of muscles.
- Delayed relaxation phases of muscles
- Painful cramps.

Diagnosis

Laboratory evaluation:
- Elevated CK in symptomatic patients
- Creatine is not elevated.
- Increased TSH with low free and total T4.
- Macrocytic anemia around 10 gm/dl
- Elevated antithyroid antibodies in autoimmune thyroiditis.

EMG: EMG shows the following features:
- Normal or low amplitude polyphasic motor unit potentials,
- Increased insertional activity
- Positive sharp waves.

Pathology: The pathological examination shows the following features:
- Atrophy, necrosis and hypertrophy of fibers.
- Inflammatory infiltrate and muscle fiber necrosis in patients with rhabdomyolysis.

Acromegalic Myopathy

GH stimulates the formation of somatomedins which are insulin like growth factors.

IGF – 1 is the most important of these and is manufactured in the liver.

Muscle protein: Synthesis is increased and protein breakdown in muscle is decreased.

Clinical Presentation

- Initial increased bulk and strength.
- Insidious onset of proximal weakness.
- Fatigue and exercise intolerance.
- Muscle wasting is minimal.

Diagnosis

Laboratory features:
- Growth hormone and IGF – 1 levels are increased.
- Lack of growth hormone suppression during glucose tolerance test.
- Levels of creatinine kinase are raised.

EMG: EMG shows the following features:
- 50% of patients have myopathic changes.
- Neuropathy is observed in 50% of patients, which may be generalized or entraptment.
- Neuropathy evolution is independent of myopathy and vice versa.

Pathology: Following features are observed on pathological examination:
- Type II fiber necrosis
- Increased muscle glycogen.

Hypopituitarism

Etiology

- Pituitary tumors
- Meningioma
- Head trauma
- Thrombophlebitis
- Cysts.

Clinical Presentation

- Severe weakness: Muscle manifestations are due to reduction of thyroid hormone, or growth hormone.
- Fatigue
- Dwarfism
- Poor muscle development.

Hyperparathyroidism

General features:

- Proximal muscle weakness, wasting and cramps
- Stiffness
- Increased tendon reflexes.

Diagnosis

Laboratory investigations:

- Elevated levels of alkaline phosphatase and calcium.
- Elevated PTH levels.

EMG:

- Decreased muscle action potentials.
- Increased polyphasic potentials without spontaneous activity.

Pathology:
- Type II fiber atrophy
- Focal areas of atrophy with polymorphonuclear cell infiltrate.

Hypoparathyroidism

Clinical Presentation

- Proximal muscle weakness which may be mild.

Diagnosis

Laboratory features:
Decreased serum calcium and phosphate levels.

EMG: EMG shows spontaneous or repetitive firing.

Pathology: Pathological examination shows the following features:
- Slight atrophy
- Decreased glycogen phosphorylase activation.

Electrolyte Disorders

- Hypokalemia, or hyperkalemia can produce myopathy.
- Insidious muscle weakness developing over days.
- Cramps.
- No cognitive or sensory disturbance.

Diagnosis

EMG:
- Myopathic changes
- Occasional changes of muscle irritability.

Pathology: Pathological examination shows the following features:

- Except for multiple vacuoles in muscles, which can be seen in other diseases like SLE, alcoholic myopathy, etc. no specific changes are seen.
- Important clinical point for myopathy due to hyperkalemia is rapid onset of weakness affecting legs; weakness may also spread to arms or may mimic GBS.
- Absent DTRS.
- Cranial nerves are spared.

DISEASES OF MUSCLE AND THE MUSCLE ENDPLATE

Myasthenia Gravis

Myasthenia gravis was the first neurological disease to be clearly identified as being due to an autoimmune disorder.

For a long-time its association with thymus was known. This association was either in the form of presence of thymus or in those patients where there was no tumor yet.

Many young female patients benefited from thymectomy. Later steroids were shown to be of benefit and in more recent times antibodies to muscle endplate at neuromuscular junction (Fig. 3.2) has led to immunosuppressive treatment.

There are two sites and two types of antibodies. One site is at the acetylcholine receptor site as occurs in classical myasthenia gravis and other is against the voltage gated calcium channels of the presynaptic terminal.

The end result in both cases is partial failure of neuromuscular transmission.

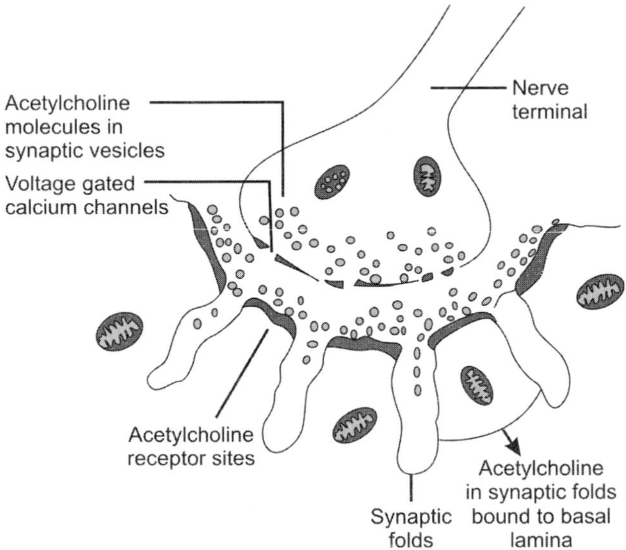

Fig. 3.2: The neuromuscular junction

Clinical features: Myasthenia gravis (Acquired and congenital).

General Features

- Incidence is 4/1,000,000
- Prevalence 0.5-5/1,00,000
- Peak incidence 25-30 years of age
- Sex females more than males.

Clinical Presentation

- Subacute onset
- Ptosis of one eyelid
- Variable symptoms.

- Proximal muscle weakness of lower extremities greater than upper extremities.
- Weakness may increase during the day.
- Specific muscle groups may show signs of fatigue on exercise. This may involve chewing, swallowing, holding the head up.
- 15% of patients it is purely ocular involvement.
- Factors which aggravate weakness include exercise, heat, stress, pregnancy, menstrual history, hypokalemia, hypo and hyperthyroidism and viral infection.
- 50% of patients present with ptosis and diplopia.
- Bulbar complaints occur in 20% of patients.

Clinical Examination

- Ptosis is usually asymmetrical
- Normal pupils
- III, IV, V nerve weakness
- Lower facial weakness
- Sluggish gag reflex
- Nasal speech
- Difficulty in swallowing fluids
- Neck flexor and extensor weakness
- Respiratory muscle weakness may be part of generalized weakness or may occur as an isolated sign.
- Isolated bulbar weakness occurs and many a times there may be difficulty in weaning the patients off the respirator.

Diagnosis

EMG: EMG evaluation shows the following features:

Jolly response is positive in 85% of patients with generalized MG.

Decrement response which may be as low as 10%.

Maximal contraction of the muscle for 30-60 seconds abolishes the decrement (post-teranic potential) for 120 seconds after the exercise.

The decrement is increased (posttetanic potentials) for 120-240 seconds following exercise.

Single fiber EMG

- Single fiber EMG is abnormal in 95-100% of MG patients.
- Jitter (latency variability between single muscle fiber potential) innervated by same axon is increased in MG.
- Blocking (absence of second muscle fiber potential) may be noted.

Laboratory evaluation:

Antibodies to acetylcholine receptor:

1. Positive in 85-90% of patients with generalized MG.
2. Positive in 30-40% of patients with ocular MG.

CT scan chest: To evaluate for the presence of thymic tumor.

Serum antibodies: To muscle specific receptor tyrosine kinase (MUSK):

- Found in generalized sero negative MG patients; 20% of all MG patients.
- All patients tested seronegative for MUSK were women.

EMG: EMG may be myopathic with chronic denervation.

Clinical Features

- Not specific nevertheless in these patients, neck, shoulder and respiratory weakness is common.
- Response to choline esterase inhibitors is variable.

Myasthenia Gravis due to Decreased Response to Acetylcholine

Fast Channel Syndromes

- Three syndromes have been described
- The cardinal feature of all three syndromes is that they have brief channel openings.
- Response to pyridostigmine; 3-4 diaminopyridine
- There is mutation of extracellular domain of the delta submitunit (delta P/2IL).
- Due to these changes in alpha and beta chain subunits, the gate may open slowly and may close rapidly.

Slow Channel Syndrome

- In this group of syndrome designated as Slow channel syndrome, there is prolonged opening of AChR
- It shows autosomal dominant inheritance pattern.
- *EMG:* Repetitive muscle action potentials and endplate potentials demonstrate staircase summation and depolarization block.

LAMBERT-EATON MYASTHENIC SYNDROME (LEMS)

General Features

- Presynaptic failure to release acetylcholine packets.
- Autoimmune etiology is suggested by antibodies to various organs, such as thyroid in 25% of cases.
- Improvement after plasma exchange and immunosuppressant therapy.

- Small lung cell cancer is present in 60% of patients.
- Type I fiber loss in muscle biopsy and progressive atrophy.

Clinical Presentation

- Incidence greater than 50 years
- Associated with small cell carcinoma of lungs.
- Leg weakness, proximal > distal
- Pain and dysesthesia may be present
- Muscle strength may seem to increase after voluntary contraction followed by fatigue.
- Cranial nerves less commonly affected.
- Respiratory failure occurs.

Diagnosis

EMG: Shows the following features:
- Amplitude of the resting MAP (Muscle action potential) induced by supramaximal stimulation is reduced.
- Slow repetitive maximal nerve stimulation less than 10 seconds causes a further decrement.
- Single fiber EMG demonstrated abnormal firing and blocking.

Laboratory features:
- Voltage gated calcium channel antibodies present in 80% of patients.

Management

Management is more or less same to that of classical myasthenia gravis except that if there is no response to neostigmine, acetylcholine release may be improved by the use of 3,4-diaminopyridine 10-20 mg, QDS. Most patients, however, need steroids and immunosuppressant drug azathioprine.

Drugs used in MG are described below:

Anticholinergic drugs:

- They must be used with caution as they tend to produce, cramps, sweating, tachycardia, blurring of vision, etc.
- Neostigmine in the dose of 15-30 mg, 4 hourly is quick acting and has a short duration of action.
- Pyridostigmine in the dose of 30-120 mg, 6-8 hourly is longer lasting, and is best supplemented with prostigmine.

Steroids

- With steroids like prednisolone, dose adjustment is important.
- Young female patients may require more than 60-120 mg (1-1.5 mg/kg) on alternate days to be effective.
- Elderly male patients may respond to doses as low as 2.5-5 mg, TDS.

Immunosuppression

- Azathioprine has become a standard immunosuppressive drug in a dose range of 25-50 mg, TDS (2.5 mg/kg/per day).
- Increase in red cell diameter to between 105-110 mm can be considered as a good parameter for adjustment of the dose.
- Hematological parameters must be regularly monitored. Sometimes the patients on azathioprine may take months to show improvement.
- In addition to immunosuppression, plasmapharesis and immunoglobulins are also used in management of myasthenia gravis.

Drugs Affecting the Neuromuscular Junction

A number of drugs may cause weakness and paralysis by affecting the neuromuscular junction and the muscle itself. They act in following ways:

a. Blocking NMJ by temporarily affecting NMJ and producing myasthenia like syndrome
b. Unmasking previous NMJ abnormality
c. Delays recovery after the use of NMJ blocking agents during anesthesia.

Antibiotics Aminoglycosides

- Streptomycin
- Neomycin
- Tobramycin
- Gentamicin.

Anticonvulsants

- Phenytoin may affect the NMJ by a membrane stabilizing effect.
- B-blockers: Block ion pump mechanisms in muscle membrane.
- Calcium blocking agents often cause muscle cramps.
- Steroids paradoxically steroids may worsen myasthenia in earlier stages of their use in MG. Long-term they may damage type 2b muscle fibers and cause myopathy.
- Lithium: Affects NMJ by depleting sodium from nerve terminals and interfering with ion pump mechanism at the presynaptic level.
- D-penicillamine used in treatment of Wilson's disease, cystinuria causes production of anti-acetylcholine antibodies giving rise to similar picture as seen in MG.

- Organophosphates used as insecticides block NMJ by irreversible inactivation of acetylcholinesterase producing deporalizing blockade.

Botulinum Toxin

- Toxin binds to voltage gated calcium channels of the presynaptic membrane causing progressive fatal paralysis
- Botulism occurs following wound infection with *Clostridium botulinum* and classically as a result of ingestion of the toxin produced by the bacteria in inadequately preserved foods.

Snake Venoms

- Two sites: Causing NMJ blocking – Presynaptic and Postsynaptic.
- Presynaptic acting toxins are lethal and postsynaptic acting toxins are less lethal the former are phospholipases and the latter are polypeptides.

Tetanus

Tetanus occurs worldwide, about 25% from occupational exposure.

Clostridium tetani

Toxin transported to both the sensory neurons of the dorsal root ganglia and archenteric neurons.

Clinical Features

- Rigidity of masseters
- Generalized spasms with opisthotonos

- No loss of consciousness
- Painful muscles with increased reflexes.

Cephalic Tetanus

- Lower cranial nerves are involved
- Facial weakness
- Dysphagia
- Ophthalmoplegia
- Source: Middle ear infection
- The toxin acts on the muscles or motor nerve endings as well as on the spinal cord and brainstem.

Neonatal Tetanus

- Source of infection: Infected umbilical stump
- Weakness and inability to suck during the second weeks of life.

EMG

- Continuous and excessive motor unit activity
- Normal nerve conduction studies
- Absent silent period from affected muscles.

4 Diseases of Anterior Horn Cell

Although there is a fair degree of overlap between anterior horn cells; roots and nerves; and muscle diseases: Anterior horn cell disease is considered as a separate entity. This is especially so since there has been better understanding of anterior horn cells anatomically, physiologically and as a relay station between spinal cord, motor system and peripheral nervous system. Besides, there is a wide variation available

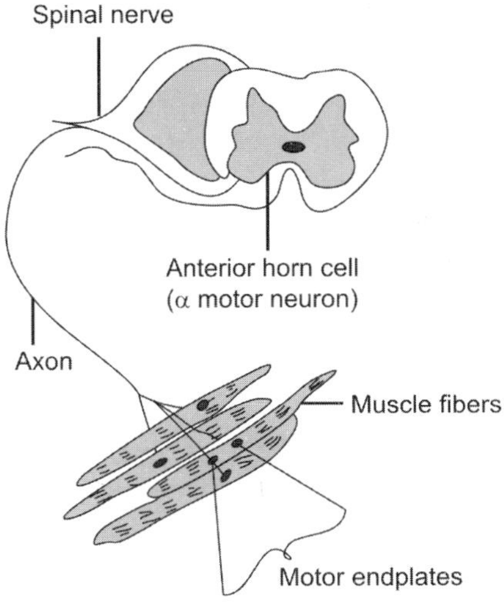

Fig. 4.1: A motor unit comprising of alpha motor neuron, spinal nerve and muscle fibers

for genetic counseling, for instance in commonly thought of anterior horn cell disease such as amyotrophic lateral sclerosis, other primary hereditary degenerative diseases which are also associated with ALS and anterior horn cell diseases. This differentiation is of prognostic importance. In the future, there is increased likelihood for discovery and availability of better treatment options due to improved understanding of autoimmune disease mechanism, attack on the motor neurons, and muscles and their related genes. Figure 4.1 depicts a motor unit comprising of alpha motor neuron, spinal nerve and muscle fibers.

INHERITED ANTERIOR HORN CELL DISEASE

Werdnig-Hoffmann Disease (Infantile Spinal Muscular Atrophy)

It is inherited as an autosomal recessive disease. It begins *in utero* and the mother may be aware of poor fetal movements in the third trimester of pregnancy. The child at birth may be 'floppy' with - complete hypotonia of limbs and difficulty in breathing and feeding. There usually is areflexia. Fasciculations may not be frankly seen. Respiratory paralysis occurs early and is the cause of death in most cases.
The child usually dies in the first year of life.

Intermediate forms do occur and usually the child develops normally till 1 year of age. The disease starts manifesting usually when the child starts walking. Tongue wasting and fasciculations appear. There is no respiratory muscle paralysis and the disease appears to be arrested.

Kugelberg-Welander Syndrome (Juvenile Spinal Muscular Atrophy)

Clinical Features

- It may be autosomal recessive or autosomal dominant.
- Genes linked to chromosome 5.
- Onset occurs early in childhood or late teens.
- Proximal muscles are involved.
- There may be clear cut fasciculations, but less of wasting.
- There are no pyramidal signs.
- No reflex change and the plantars are flexors.
- Weakness is of proximal lower limb muscles, the pelvic girdle being earliest affected.
- The gait may be waddling type and often Duchenne and Becker type of dystrophies are considered in the diagnosis.
- The lifespan is normal, though most patients eventually need a wheelchair.
- Shoulder girdle muscles are affected at later stage.
- Bulbar muscle involvement does not occur.

Diagnosis

Laboratory evaluation: Creatinine kinase (CK) may be raised up to 10 times the normal value.

EMG: EMG shows the following features:
- Positive sharp waves, and reduced interference pattern.
- No muscle action potential.
- Motor nerve conduction velocity is normal.

Differential Diagnosis

It is important to mention differential diagnosis of Kugelberg-Welander disease which includes the following:

- Duchenne muscular dystrophy
- Becker's muscular dystrophy.

The hallmark of KW disease is presence of fasciculations. In DMD and BMD there are no fasciculations. The CK is very much higher in dystrophies mentioned.

Congenital myopathies are associated with extraocular muscle paralysis, cardiac defects and dysmorphisms, which differentiate them from spinal muscular atrophy. On EMG, denervation is seen in all forms of spinal muscular atrophies. Fasciculations are common. Sural nerve action potentials are normal and motor nerve conduction velocities are normal.

SPINAL MUSCULAR ATROPHIES NOT LINKED TO CHROMOSOME 5Q

Late Onset Tay-Sachs Disease

- Autosomal recessive inheritance
- Accumulation of GM2 ganglioside in neurons, resulting from decrease of hexosaminidase, a lysosomal enzyme
- The disease results due to dysfunction of alpha and beta chain on the gene of either Chromosome 5 or 15.

Clinical Features

- Age of onset is usually second decade of life.
- Dysarthria and truncal ataxia may precede limb weakness.
- Prominent feature is lower motor neuron involvement.
- Associated features include psychosis, dementia, and dystonia.

Diagnosis

EMG evaluation: The EMG shows the following features:

- Neurogenic.
- Normal motor nerve conduction velocity.
- Normal sensory nerve conduction velocity.

Monomelic Amyotrophy (Hirayama's Disease)

- Worldwide distribution. Most patients are from Japan and India.
- There are two mechanisms of disease: (a) Spinal cord ischemia, (b) Abnormal cervical ligaments.

Clinical Features

- A sporadic disease.
- Unilateral weakness and atrophy of intrinsic hand muscles, gradual progression over 3 years then stops.
- There may be fine tremors in the extended fingers of affected hands.
- No upper motor neuron signs.
- Normal reflexes and normal sensations.

Diagnosis

Laboratory evaluation: On laboratory investigations, the following abnormalities are seen:

- Elevated CK.
- Normal blood chemistries and CSF.

EMG: The EMG shows the following features:

- Motor nerve conduction is normal.
- Preserved sural nerve action potentials.
- Signs of denervation are seen in most patients.
- Contralateral limb may also show EMG abnormalities.

MRI: Cervical and upper thoracic cord atrophy.

INFECTIVE VENTRAL HORN DISEASE

Acute Anterior Poliomyelitis

- Infections most commonly occur in late summers.
- Transmitted by fecal – oral route.
- Pharyngeal spread occurs during epidemics.
- It has become rare disease in the developed world due to vaccination, nevertheless yearly epidemics do occur.
- Disease usually occurs in the non-immune individuals traveling to the tropics and other less sanitary areas of the world.
- Polio remains a major risk as virus is transmitted by fecal-oral soiling of drinking water.

Clinical Features

- Aseptic meningitis which in 1% of cases may go on to become fatal paralytic poliomyelitis.
- It usually starts after an acute viral respiratory tract infection.
- There may be severe muscle pains, painful paresthesiae, with headache and photophobia.
- A week later, rapid weakness develops with severe cramps and fasciculations in the affected muscles.
- The muscles affected are in the lumbar and cervicothoracic regions which are supplied by same motor pools so a large group of muscles are affected.
- With affectation of respiratory muscles - respiratory care by artificial respiratory may be necessary. In this particular situation as recovery occurs, only few muscles may be left which remain permanently weak giving rise to localized abnormality.

- Burnt out or 'old polio' may be seen with manifestations such as atrophy and weakness of group of muscles with absent local reflexes. There may be involvement of autonomic nervous system giving rise to vasomotor changes such as cold, clammy, and swollen extremities.
- In these cases of 'old polio' there is higher risk of motor neuron disease. It may occur 30-40 years after poliomyelitis affectation and is thought to be due to death in those ventral horn cells which had recovered during the initial recovery stage of polio illness.
- Intrinsic hand muscle affectation is rare in polio. If subsequently one finds brisk reflexes, marked wasting and fasciculations in intrinsic muscles of the hand, it points to new pathology in 'old polio' such as motor neuron disease.
- In the legs, vasomotor changes are predominant features, with cold, puffy, purple limbs and the weakness is proximal and patchy. If at a later stage, brisk reflexes and extensor plantar responses are seen in the same patient this is the clue to development of new pathology as motor neuron disease.
- Many a times, a situation may arise when the anterior compartment muscles of both legs are weak and remain so over many years. So extensor plantar response cannot be elicited. In the same situation if deep tendon reflexes are lost in the polio illness they cannot be brisk even though a new pathology like motor neuron disease manifests itself for the first-time in the same 'old polio' patient. Here we have to rely on weakness, wasting, often fasiculations in group of muscles, typical of pyramidal disease. Specific group of muscles are: (1) in the upper limbs shoulder abductors, the elbow extensors, wrist extensors; (2) in the legs, hip flexors, knee flexors (Hamstrings) and dorsiflexors of the foot.

Diagnosis

Laboratory evaluation:

Evaluation of CSF shows the following features:

- Polymorphonuclear leucocytosis occurs early.
- Proteins are elevated (100 -300 mg/dl).
- Sugar normal.
- Virus is isolated from CSF, stools, urine.

EMG: Electromyography is of no diagnostic importance particularly when new pathology as motor neuron disease occurs in 'old polio' cases. The following features may be seen:

- Chronic partial denervation
- Prolonged giant motor units in the greatly reduced interference pattern are seen.
- Fasciculation and fibrillation are absent.

TOXIC ANTERIOR HORN CELL DISEASE

- Toxic substances like tri-ortho-cresyl phosphate may affect the anterior horn cells.
- 'Jamaica ginger' a component of illicit liquor during prohibition in USA caused outbreak of the disease.
- Aviation oil containing TOCP was sold as cooking oil in Morocco which caused an epidemic of poisoning.
- Tick paralysis: Tick gets embedded in skin in the scalp or neck and these ticks causing fever and paralysis are particularly found in Rocky Mountains of Canada and USA and also in Balkan states. Full clinical picture consists of:
  - Facial paresthesiae
  - Difficulty in swallowing
  - Ascending paralysis.

Electrical Injury

Clinical Features

- The source of the current is usually from household circuits, high voltage line or lightening.
- These may cause severe burns and cardiac arrest.
- The electric current passes down corticospinal tract and bladder pathways. Weakness of muscles and atrophy of muscles begins at the site of injury and may spread contralaterally.
- Bulbar signs and upper motor neuron weakness occurs.

Postradiation Motor Neuron Syndrome

- Delayed occurrence after X – RT
  - 3000 rads to cervical spine
  - 5000 rads to lumbosacral spine.
- Occurs months or years after treatment.
- There is atrophy and fasciculation of muscles. Sensations are normal.
- Bladder is not involved.
- Weakness stabilizes over years but may progress.
- When the radiation is given to neck or head exceeding >3000 rads, lower cranial nerves may be involved and sometimes carotid artery is damaged giving rise to stroke.

EMG: EMG evaluation shows the following features:

- Myokemic discharges
- Fibrillation potentials are present in the lower extremities.

Laboratory evaluation: Laboratory evaluation shows the following features:

- CSF is normal
- Protein is raised.

Motor Neuron Disease

Five percent of patients of MND have positive family history. The pattern of inheritance indicates autosomal dominant gene. Further analysis of gene indicates defect in the enzyme superoxide dismutase on chromosome 21.

Amyotrophic Lateral Sclerosis

General Features

- Incidence varies from 0.2 to 2.4 per 100,000 people in the world.
- Prevalence rate is between 0.8 and 7.4 per 100,000 people.
- Risk factor is the age; death usually occurs between 55-75 years.
- Male to female ratio is 1.5-2.5
- 50% die within 3 years of diagnosis
- 75% die within 5 years of diagnosis
- 10% live longer than 10 years.
- 90% of cases of ALS are sporadic.

Clinical Features

- Atrophy of intrinsic hand muscles: Pattern may be; (a) First dorsal interosseous; (b) 4th-5th fingers weakness and wasting.
- Atrophy and fasciculation in a particular muscle group with increased reflexes.
- Bulbar distribution weakness.
- Foot drop, wrist drop.
- Spasticity and hypereflexia are invariably present.

Primary Lateral Sclerosis

- Lower motor neuron not involved.
- Age of onset between 50 and 55 years.
- Progress occurs slowly.
- Clinical presentation may be in form of spastic paraparesis, bilateral Babinski's sign and Hoffmann's sign.
- Pseudobulbar palsy
- Cognition is affected.

Progressive Muscular Atrophy

Rare variant of MND occurs in 2.5% of patients.

Slow progression better outcome in terms of survival than ALS A pure Lower Motor Neuron Disease.

Closet differential diagnosis is spinal muscular atrophy.

Clinical feature distal wasting and weakness which may affect arm or leg.

EMG: EMG shows chronic denervation.

Gum Parkinsonian ALS Dementia Complex

- Endemicity: Western Pacific; Kii peninsula of Japan; West New Guinea
- Genetics: No gene has been identified
- Clinical feature: Parkinsonism Akinetic rigid variety; facial (mouth) dystonia; and severe dementia.

5 Spinal Cord

ANATOMY OF SPINAL CORD

The spinal cord is approximately 45 cm long and this extends from top of C1 vertebra to the lower part of L1 vertebra.

The spinal cord at birth may be as low as L3 vertebra and by the age of 10 years it reaches to the position of bottom of L1 vertebra. It is not cylindrical in the true sense of the definition having enlargements at cervical and lumbar levels. This is important to note as these are the areas wherein there is concentration of motor pools that supply the arms and the legs and therefore there is considerable enlargement of the gray matter in these areas. Anatomical boundaries are from C3 – T2 and from L1 – to S3. The upper end of spinal cord maintains its continuity with medulla oblongata and at the lower end the conus medullaris becomes the filum terminale. The spinal cord in its entire length is surrounded by dura mater which is separated from inner covering of the spinal cord arachnoid mater and this leaves a potential space called subdural space between the Dura and the arachnoid. The arachnoid is separated from the spinal cord by pia mater which forms the inner covering of the spinal cord and the nerve roots and the space between the arachnoid and the pia is the subarachnoid space which contains the cerebrospinal fluid.

The space between L2 and S2 contains only lumbar, sacral and coccygeal nerve roots and this constitutes the cauda equina. It is from this space that cerebrospinal fluid is drawn without injuring the spinal cord which ends at L2 and the dural sac at S2.

Internal Structure of the Spinal Cord

Transverse sections of spinal cord at different levels is shown in Figure 5.1. The central gray matter consists of an H-shaped area present at all levels. At midline it is joined by the gray commissure within which lies the small central canal.

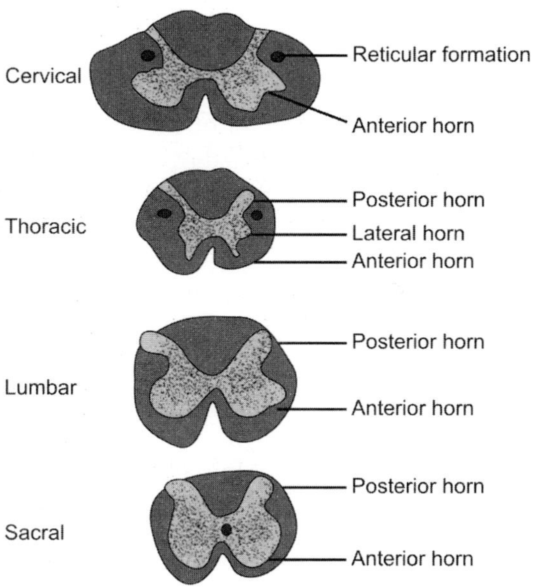

Fig. 5.1: Transverse sections of spinal cord at different levels

The gray matter is referred to as the anterior and posterior columns.

The anterior gray column contains the large cells of the alpha motor neurons and smaller motor neurons of gamma fibers. These cells are grouped into motor neuron pools which control group of muscles having similar action being called flexors and extensors.

The posterior lateral gray matter comprises of the dorsal root entry zone, cell bodies and fibers of Lissauer's tract, the substantia gelatinosa and the dorsal funicular gray matter containing nuclear masses at different levels. The lower end of spinal cord at S2 S3 S4 contains preganglionic parasympathetic cells of the pelvic splanchanic nerves.

EMBRYOLOGY

Notochord develops by the end of 15 days as endodermal cells which have migrated to form the primitive streak. By day 21, neurenteric canal is formed by fusion of notochord with endoderm.

If neurenteric canal persists, each half of vertebral body tries to form a complete vertebra. By day 28, folding of the notochord forms a tube. Somites are formed by segmentation of mesoderm by 21 days and the process is complete by day 35. In total, there are 42 somites.

Formation of brain and spinal cord occurs by formation of neural plate from the center of the cells. The lateral margins join the midline; the fusion begins at third and fourth somites.

The anterior neuropore closes at 24 days and posterior neuropore at 26 days.

The pia-arachnoid mater, dorsal root ganglia, Schwann cells of the peripheral nerves, the autonomic ganglia, the skin tissue, the chromaffin tissue and the cartilage in the branchial arches are formed by the neural crest.

Cells of neural crest also form the spinal ganglia down to L1 – 2 level.

However, lower portion extending from lumbar, sacral and coccygeal cord are formed at a later stage by process of canalization. The distal portion of the neural tube atrophies forming the filum terminale.

It is also important to make a brief mention of the development of the vertebral column.

The notochord is surrounded by cells from the mesoderm which eventually become the vertebra and intervertebral disc. The process begins at the cervical region and extends both upwards and downwards. This process starts around day 23 with intervening phases termed as cartilaginous phase, which begins at day 40. Final ossification starts between 20-24 weeks beginning at lower thoracic and upper lumbar vertebra and extending first downwards towards the tail then towards the head.

Development of the Brain

Development of the brain is also considered here as some of the cranial anomalies are also associated with spinal anomalies. At 24 days, the neural tube becomes fully closed and three main parts are formed, i.e. forebrain, midbrain and hindbrain.

The neural crest only extends as far as the midbrain and contributes to the formation of cranial nerves III-XII.

The I and II nerves develop as direct extension of the forebrain with the flexure of the embryo important flexures of the three main parts occur. The first flexion occurs between cervical cord and the midbrain the cephalic between the forebrain and the midbrain and the growth of the cerebral hemisphere envelops what is called the brainstem. The pontine flexure occurring at the mid – hindbrain forms the fourth ventricle. This occurs at 30 and 36 days.

A remnant of the central cavity of the forebrain becomes divided into two lateral ventricles during rapid development of cerebral hemispheres and the midline into third ventricle. The third ventricle is separated into two halves by two layers of pia mater with a potential space between them called cavum septum pellucidum which is filled with cerebrospinal fluid.

Two commissures, anterior and posterior and corpus callosum join two cerebral hemispheres.

Anterior commissure links olfactory bulbs and temporal lobes. All other areas are linked by corpus callosum. At 56 days, the anterior roof of the fourth ventricle thickens to become the rhombic lip which then rapidly enlarges to form the cerebellum. The roof plate of the fourth ventricle becomes thinner and perforates to allow CSF to communicate with the subarachnoid space through the foramina of Luschke and Magendie's.

BLOOD SUPPLY OF SPINAL CORD

The spinal cord is supplied principally by two spinal arteries: (1) Anterior spinal artery; (2) Posterior spinal artery (Figs 5.2A and B).

There is great degree of anastomosis between the branches of the two main arteries.

The central area is supplied by the sulcal arteries which are branches of anterior spinal arteries. Other branches of anterior spinal arteries are circumferential arteries.

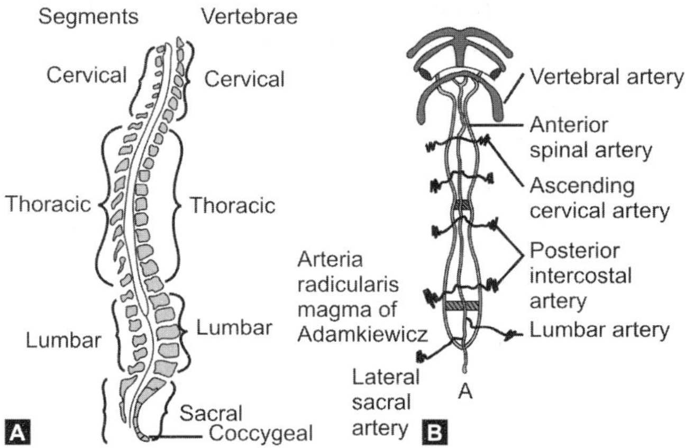

Figs 5.2A and B: (A) The spinal segments and their corresponding vertebral levels, (B) Arterial supply of the spinal cord

The anterior spinal artery arises from the vertebral arteries in the foramen magnum as two vessels that join to become a single vessel opposite odontoid peg.

There is fair degree of replenishment of the anterior spinal artery at cervical and thoracic region. One important artery is the "**Artery of Adamkiewicz",** which arises from intercostal artery.

The lower spinal cord and nerve roots of the cauda equina are supplied by a variable vessel entering the canal on one of the upper lumbar roots.

PHYSIOLOGY OF THE SPINAL CORD

The physiological principles concerning spinal cord are considered only in terms of its afferent pathway.

Ascending paths in the brainstem, motor projections from the cortex and brainstem to the spinal motor neuron:

Cutaneous sensibility: The fibers subserving skin, pain, temperature and a part of those for touch end round the cells of the dorsal horn of gray matter. The fibers which arise here cross to ventrolateral columns of white matter of the opposite side to constitute the spinothalamic tract.

The tract consists of two divisions a lateral one, carrying pain and temperature fibers and a ventral one carrying touch fibers. The spinothalamic tract also contains pain fibers from muscles and related structures and viscera. Fibers subserving sexual and bladder sensations, fibers subserving tickle, itch and muscular fatigue, and some of the fibers for touch pass into the dorsal columns of the same side.

The crossing of spinothalamic fibers takes place round the central canal of the spinal cord in the gray commissure. In the lower level of spinal cord these fibers cross transversely in the segment from which they arise. In the higher levels of the cord this crossing becomes increasingly oblique. In the thoracic region it occupies two or three segments, in the cervical region four or five segments.

Fibers for pain cross transversely at all levels, those for touch most obliquely those for temperature occupy an intermediate position.

Deep sensibility: The fibers carrying impulses from deep structures end in three ways.

1. Some end round Clarke's column of cells at base of the dorsal horn, chiefly in the thoracic and upper lumbar region. Two tracts: Dorsocerebellar tract and ventral spinocerebellar tract arise from this column. They convey impulses from the muscles, tendons and joints to the

cerebellum. Cerebellum depends upon integrity of these two columns whereby it receives impulses from deeper structures such as muscles, tendons, joints and thus maintains posture and coordinates functions of the muscles.

2. Some end in the spinal gray matter or pass up to the brainstem nuclei, e.g. vestibular, reticular nuclei or red nucleus and are concerned with reflex posture and reflex movements.
3. The other fibers from the deep structures pass up directly in the dorsal columns of the spinal cord.

In the cervical region, the dorsal columns are divided by a septum the medial column, the funiculus gracilis and the lateral column, the funiculus cuneatus.

a. The funiculus gracilis arises from ganglion cells of dorsal nerve roots which carry afferent impulses from the lower limbs and the lower half of the trunk.

   Every fiber, as it enters the dorsal columns of the cord comes to lie close to the medial side of the dorsal horn. As it is ascends the cord, it is gradually displaced medially by fibers which enter at higher levels. The tract ends in the nucleus gracilis in the medulla.
b. The funiculus cuneatus arises from ganglion cells of the dorsal nerve supplying the upper limbs and upper half of the trunk. It occupies the lateral part of the dorsal column of white matter and ends in the nucleus cuneatus in the medulla.

A further relay of fibers from these medullary nuclei passes to the thalamus and thence to the sensory cortex. There, the impulses give rise to sensations about the position of the limbs in space and the direction and extent of movements whether passive or active.

Ascending Paths in the Brainstem

From the gracile and cuneate nuclei, a fresh relay of fibers sweeps ventrally across the midline to form the medial lemniscus which lies near the midline dorsal to the pyramid.

These carry impulses from joint receptors, from touch receptors and from pacinian corpuscles.

Spinothalamic Tract

The fibers which carry impulses from pain and temperature receptors remain on the surface of the medulla lateral to the olivary nucleus where they mingle with spinocerebellar tract.

All fibers ultimately join the medial lemniscus and carry all impulses from the skin and muscles of the opposite side of the body below the head.

Cranial Nerves

The fifth nerve after receiving impulses ends in the principal sensory nucleus of the pons and in the long descending root and adjacent gray matter which extends down to the upper cervical cord.

A fresh relay of fibers after crossing the midline from this long gray matter enters the medial lemniscus.

Fibers of the ophthalmic division of the fifth nerve end in the lowest part of the spinal part of the descending root, the maxillary division ends in the middle part of the root, the superior part of the nucleus receives mandibular division of the nerve.

Thus, the face is represented 'upside down' in the nucleus.

The medial lemniscus also receive fibers from other sensory cranial nerve nuclei, vagus, the dorsal nuclei of the ninth and seventh nerves and from the vestibular division of the eighth nerve.

The fibers from the medial lemniscus ascend the brainstem and give off many collaterals to the adjacent neurons of the reticular system.

Motor Projections from the Cortex and Brainstem to the Spinal Motor Neurons

Upper motor neurons are those spinal motor neurons which receive impulses from the cortex and the brainstem. These are termed as pyramidal and extrapyramidal tracts.

Voluntary movement is effected by impulses which descend over these upper motor neurons to excite the spinal motor neurons. The state of excitability of these motor neurons is profoundly modified by such supraspinal influences, thus muscle tone although due to spinal reflexes can be modified by both facilitatory and inhibitory upper motor neurons.

DISEASES OF SPINAL CORD

The disease affectation of the spinal cord is considered under following headings and is discussed in order of their clinical importance.

- Vascular
- Infective
- Tumors
- Demyelinating
- Congenital defects
- Vertebral column – Bony disease
- Trauma
- Spastic paraplegias
- Nutritional

SPINAL CORD TRAUMA

The majority of serious spinal injuries occur in the dorsal area, particularly between T-6 and T12. The mobility of cervical and lumbar spine protect these areas from damage. In the absence of known diseases of vertebra—primary osteoporosis, metastasis, steroid use, osteoporosis secondary to radiation, a considerable degree of force is required to damage the spinal cord either due to fracture of the vertebra and or fracture dislocation.

The Mechanisms of Injuries

Sudden violent flexion of the neck (fracture of the cervical vertebra)

- Anterior compression fracture of the vertebral bodies
- Facet joint dislocation
- Rupture of the longitudinal and interspinous ligaments.
  - Severe compression injury.
  - Due to falls affecting thoracic lumbar areas.
  - Rotational injury usually from facet dislocation.
  - Hyperextension of the neck resulting in fracture of the posterior elements possibly due to spondylolisthesis at the affected levels.

Parenchymatous Cord Trauma Cases

General Considerations

- Motor vehicle accidents.
- Sport injuries
- Gunshot wounds
- The incidence in industrialized countries and India has leveled off to similar peak.

- Incidence: 30-40/100,000 population
- Prevalence: 900/100,000 population
- Over 70% of patients are between the age of 20-35 years with male to female ratio being 3:1.
- Over 30-40% of population is in the age group of 55-60 years.
- These injuries occur throughout the year but may show increased peak in summer months and winter months in different regions of the world.

Patterns of Parenchymatous Spinal Cord Damage

- Cord concussion
- Spinal shock
- Complete cord transection (rare)
- Often seen as incomplete cord compression, clinically manifesting as:
  - Brown-Séquard's syndrome
  - Central cord syndrome
  - Anterior cord syndrome
  - Posterior cord syndrome.

Associated Injuries

- To the vertebral arteries resulting in brainstem infarction.
- To the cauda equina which may be complete or partial.

Spinal Concussion

Transient neurological symptoms occur with full recovery over minutes to hours. The signs are below the level of the injury.

Spinal Shock

- Complete flaccid paralysis below the level of the lesion.
- Loss of sensation below the level of the lesion.

- Incontinence of bladder and bowel.
- Areflexia below the level of the lesion.
- Extensor plantar.
- Areflexia, and hypotonia which may change to hyperreflexia usually by 4-6 weeks.

As the recovery is slow and many a times very little recovery occurs in motor and sensory system leaving chronic neurological deficit, autonomic disturbances may dominate the picture resulting in :

- Hypertension
- Hyperhidrosis
- Severe headache
- Seizures.

Brown-Séquard's Syndrome

- Classical picture is that of signs pointing to hemisection of the cord.
- Ipsilateral paralysis below the level of the lesion.
- Ipsilateral loss of vibration, propioception and light touch.
- Contralateral loss of pain and temperature sensibility.
- Bladder and bowel functions remain intact.

Central Cord Syndrome

- Hands and arms are affected more than the legs.
- Usually there is sacral sparing and the sensory loss may be incomplete.
- Acute urinary retention occurs in 50% of patients.
- Recovery of bladder, bowel and sexual function commonly occurs.
- Pyramidal tract damage is manifested by spasticity and extensor plantars.

Due to similarity of signs seen in posterior cord damage in conditions other than trauma such as demyelinating disease, tumors, etc. the clinical features are mentioned here:

- Loss of vibration and joint sense with positive rombergism.
- The propioceptive loss may be severe to the extent that the patient may be unable to walk in the dark.
- Lhermitte's sign is present.
- Due to severe loss of postural sense, abnormal wild movements of the arms are seen.

Cauda Equina Lesion

- Acute disk protrusion
- Spinal stenosis
- Metastatic tumors
- Vertebral fractures resulting in posterior displacement of bone fragments into the spinal canal.

Clinical Features

- Motor and sensory loss is asymmetric
- Severe pain is dominant feature
- Perineal sensory anesthesiae
- Bowel and bladder disfunction
- Areflexia.

Post-traumatic Syringomyelia

In recent years it has been recognized that syringomyelic syndrome may complicate spinal cord trauma. The syringomyelic syndrome may occur anywhere between 1-15 years. A paraplegic who has stabilized may show new signs pointing to new pathology. Pain is the first symptom. Lower motor neurons signs develop in the form of wasting and weakness.

CT scan, MRI confirm the presence of syringomyelic cavity in the damaged area.

A similar syndrome after trivial cervical injury is seen wherein the damaged cervical cord may show syrinx cavity on imaging.

Thoracolumbar Injuries

In the elderly, osteoporosis is common and single crush fractures of lumbar vertebra are seen which may leave no neurological sequale. However in patients with malignancy of the prostrate or primary malignancy of the vertebra, myelomatosis, etc. spinal cord compression is common. Similarly crush fractures which can rarely give rise to cord deficit are seen in epileptics due to tonic clonic seizures.

Bladder: Micturition Disturbances

It is appropriate to discuss bladder disturbances due to spinal cord and cauda equina damage here. Few fundamental details need be understood concerning pathological changes in bladder function. During history taking, the main questions to be asked of a patient with bladder dysfunction are as follows:

1. Does he have any sense of bladder filling?
2. Can he feel the urine passing?
3. Can he stop the urine passing in midstream at will?
4. Is there leakage of urine continually or the patient suddenly passes large volume?
5. Is the patient aware of rectal disorder such as incomplete passing of stools, constipation, incontinence, etc?
6. Does the patient have potency problem?
7. Is there any numbness in the perineum?

Physiology

The bladder is an empty hollow organ of smooth muscle containing stretch receptors. Bladder contracts at the influence of parasympathetic nerves. This is called autonomic stretch reflex. A large volume is made to collect in the bladder without rise of intravesicular pressure. The parasympathetic reflex is based on the S3 roots and S3 segment of the cord.

The stretch receptors fire impulses proportional to the stretch of the bladder wall and weight of the urine.

Any inflammation or infection of the bladder results in adverse effect on the stretch receptors making them more sensitive and thus altering the normal physiology of micturition.

The basic sacral reflex arc (parasympathetic reflex) controls micturition in infancy, senility, unconsciousness, spinal cord lesions and other nervous system lesions. Voluntary control of bladder mechanism is controlled by an area in the second frontal gyrus and the main descending pathways lie in or adjacent to corticospinal tracts. The intervening pathways are in the pons and hypothalamus and exert direct physical control over the external sphincter and pelvic floor. These bring about inhibition of the conditioned reflex. **Disturbances of micturition are an early sign of spinal cord compression.**

The sympathetic outflow from T11 to L2 via the hypogastric plexus descends into the pelvis and has an inhibitory role in micturition. It relaxes the dertrusor muscles, inhibits transmission into parasympathetic ganglia, contracts the trigone and the urethra. These actions oppose the onset of micturition.

Micturition involves complete relaxation of volitional control. The external sphincter and pelvic floor relax and the local reflex is allowed to take over.

As the detrusor contracts, the bladder neck is pulled open and this combined with inhibition of weak internal sphincter allows urine to flow by a combination of rising intravesical pressure and gravity.

NEUROLOGICAL DISORDERS AFFECTING BLADDER FUNCTION

It is important that low pressure is maintained in the bladder at all times.

Small high pressure bladders are found in spinal cord disease these may lead to secondary renal damage.

Main types of neurological dysfunction are described below:

Uninhibited Bladder

This condition results due to the lesion of 2nd frontal gyrus and the pathways leading from it down to the pontine center. The lesions may present as frontal lobe tumors, normal pressure hydrocephalus, dementia, anterior communicating aneurysm or even pontine vascular and infiltrative lesion such as glioma.

Spinal Bladder

This condition may occur due to the damage to the spinal cord by trauma, cord tumor, multiple sclerosis, etc.

Clinical Presentation

- Bladder fullness may not be appreciated.
- The patient shows signs of autonomic disturbances, tachycardia, sweating, hypertension.

- Reflex emptying of the bladder may occur without warning.
- Evacuation may be incomplete.
- Associated signs of pyramidal tract damage are seen.

Autonomous Bladder (Subsacral Lesions)

This condition may occur due to the damage to motor and sensory compartments in the cauda equina or pelvis as seen in cauda equina lesions due to malignancy, spina bifida, disk lesions.

Clinical Presentation

- Dribbling incontinence
- Considerable residual urine with high infection risk
- May be associated with perineal numbness and loss of sexual function.

Sensory Bladder

Clinical features are similar to autonomous bladder and may result as a consequence of tabes dorsalis, subacute combined degeneration of the cord, multiple sclerosis, diabetes, etc.

Clinical Presentation

The retention of urine in the bladder is massive and may present as dribbling incontinence of large volumes of urine.

Residual urine with high infection rate. Evacuation incomplete.

Investigations for Bladder Dysfunction

- Biochemistry of renal functions
- Urine examination

- Measurement of residual urine after attempted complete evacuation
- Cystometrography
- Sphincter electromyography
- MRI brain and spinal cord.

Treatment for Bladder Dysfunction

- Anticholinergic drugs.
- Propantheline 15 mg TDS.
- Imipramine 10 mg TID
- Intermittent self-catheterization
- Creation of artificial bladder by specialized urinary procedures
- Permanent catheterization has infection risk, therefore silastic catheters are preferred.

DISORDERS OF POTENCY

These are four components of sexual functions in the male:

- Erection
- Secretion
- Emission
- Ejaculation

These are based on psychic influences and intact descending spinal cord pathways.

Spinal Cord Lesions

Spinal cord compression, transection of the cord, multiple sclerosis, tabes dorsalis and subacute combined degeneration of the cord, all cause impotence.

Cauda Equina Lesions

Cauda equina lesions cause impotence by causing direct damage to the reflex arc. These may be due to compression by ependymoma, cyst, lipoma, etc. The roots damaged are S5, S4, and S3.

Clinical Presentation

- Rectal pain, genital pain, micturition disturbances and loss of potency.
- Loss of ankle jerks.
- Weakness of L5 – S1 muscles.

Autonomic Nerve Lesions

1. Shy-Drager syndrome
2. Diabetes
3. Crush fracture of L1 vertebra.

This is usually associated with micturition disturbance and postural hypotension. Impotency is the earliest symptom in autonomic nerve lesions.

INFECTIVE LESIONS OF SPINAL CORD

Infections which affect the spinal cord are many. Some need to be highlighted and mentioned.

Tuberculosis is one of the commonest infective causes of spinal cord disease in acute and chronic stage.

The tuberculous process may involve the vertebral column at the cervical – Thoracic - Lumbar region.

I. It can present as Pott's disease and collapse with spinal cord compression.
II. Spinal cord infections – due to end arteritis.

III. Paravertebral abscess particularly at L1-L4 vertebra.

In the chronic stage, it can present as arachnoiditis. The clinical presentation may vary in the initial stage when only nerve roots may be involved and pain is the dominant feature with motor and sensory involvements in the distribution of that nerve root – radiculopathy. This may at the later stage progress to cord compression. By this time, the earliest presentation is of spastic weakness which may be unilateral or bilateral and symmetrical. The patient may complain of heaviness in the legs or may drag his feet. Sensory symptoms are common and may start as tingling sensation in the soles of the feet and in a matter of weeks to months may reach a higher level as the compression progresses. Micturition disturbance is a bad prognostic sign of cord compression. It may occur suddenly as urinary retention or difficulty in initiating micturition. It usually indicates progressive deterioration in cord compression.

Bacterial Infections

Commonest is *Staphylococcus aureus*.

General Considerations

There could be a presence of epidural abscess

Predisposing factors include compromised immune system; IV drug abuse; prolonged epidural anesthesia.

Clinical Features

- Severe back or neck pain.
- Occasionally there is radicular pain that may precede myelopathy.

- May present as Brown-Séquard's syndrome
- May present as sudden paralysis from spinal cord infarction.

Laboratory Evaluation

- Elevated sedimentation rate.
- *MRI evaluation*: Increased signal from the disk space on T2 weighted sequences which is the first sign of discitis.
- Enhancement of the anterior and posterior longitudanal ligaments, paraspinal muscles and the abscess.

Viral Infections with Myelitis

Myelitis may follow polio or other enterovirus infections of the anterior horn cells.

Herpes Virus

General Features

- Usually acute infections
- Sometimes there may be reactivation of the virus near the site of the original infection.
- The involved herpes viruses may be type 1 and type 2 herpes simplex virus; varicella virus; or Simian herpes B-virus.

Clinical Presentation

- Encephalitis
- Myelitis.

Diagnosis

- Increased pressure in the CSF
- Lymphocytic pleocytosis

- Glucose levels are normal or low
- Protein is elevated
- Presence of Cowdry A intranuclear inclusions.

Varicella Zoster

General Features

Latent virus may be reactivated by:
- Injury
- Immunosuppression
- Cancer
- Immunosuppressive drugs
- HIV
- Systemic illness.

Clinical Features

- T5-T2 are the affected dermatomes
- There may be myelitis involving the thoracic cord
- Associated neurologic features include postherpetic neuralgia, segmental motor atrophy and multifocal encephalitis.

Rabies

General Features

- Usual transmission is by a bite
- Reservoirs of the virus are dogs, bats, fox.
- Incubation period is between 1-2 months.

Clinical Features

- Headache
- Fever

- Paresthesia at the site of the bite.
- Severe bulbar and autonomic features.

Diagnosis

CSF: Examination may show the following features:
- High titers of neutralizing antibodies in the serum and CSF
- PCR of CSF is positive.
- Prognosis 100% fatality.
- Similar picture: May follow anti-rabies vaccination.

Polio Viruses

General Features

- Infections are most common in late summer.
- Transmission mainly occurs by fecal – oral contact.

Clinical Features

- Incubation period varies from 1-2 weeks
- Progression of illness occurs over 3-5 days
- Severe back pain – 2-3 days
- Transverse myelitis – Diaphragmatic involvement resulting in respiratory muscle paralysis, which may require artificial respiratory support.

Diagnosis

Laboratory evaluation:
- Polymorphonuclear cytosis
- Protein elevated by 100-300 mg/dl.
- Sugar is normal
- Virus isolated from CSF, stool or throat.

Retrovirus Infection

HIV binds to CD4 receptor. Infected macrophages transport the virus into the CNS. There may be occurrence of vacuolar myelopathy.

Clinical Features

- Unsteadiness of gait
- Spasticity
- Leg weakness
- Sphincter disturbances
- Babinski's sign is common.

Diagnosis

Pathology:
- Vacuolar myelopathy most prominent in dorsolateral and cervical cord.
- Myelinopathy.
- Axons are spared.

Spirochetes

Syphilis
- Caused by *T. pallidum*
- Spread occurs either by sexual contact or from mother to the child.

Clinical Features

- Lightening pains (thoracic or abdominal)
- Dorsal root ganglia involvement
- Urinary incontinence

- Romberg's sign is positive
- Argyll Robertson's pupil
- Optic atrophy
- Chorioretinitis, vasculitis
- High stepping gait.

Other Clinical Features

- Dorsal root entry zone and dorsal roots are sites of pathology.
- Compression of the cord by thickened dura.
- Anterior and posterior spinal artery occlusion.
- Endoarteritis.

Diagnosis

CSF: Serology positive
IGM and IGG antibodies are seen in the CSF.

Fugal infections

Actinomycosis

General Features

- Occurs in immunocompetent patients.
- Paravertebral abscesses, and vertebral osteomyelitis which cause spinal cord compression.
- Other infective agents causing spinal cord damage are hepatitis B virus.
- *Mycoplasma*, pneumonia, brucellosis, toxoplasmosis. Spinal cord affectation usually forms part of general picture of CNS involvement.

CONGENITAL ANOMALIES OF SPINAL CORD

Anomalies of spinal cord development which give rise to spinal cord compression and other clinical features discussed here are.

A. **Failure of neural tube closure** which is associated with skeletal modeling defects that occur around a malformed neural tube. These include:
   1. Anencephaly
   2. Meningomyelocele
   3. Cranioschisis.

B. **Bony defects due to axial mesodermal development** without a persistent open neural tube.
   These are:
   1. Encephaloceles
   2. Meningoceles
   3. Spinal bifida
   4. Diastematomyelia

In the defects no 3 and 4, the skin is covered.

Craniorachisis

- Dysraphism
- Brain and spinal cord are exposed to CSF.

Clinical Features

Necrosis degeneration and angioma like formation of the cord.

Myelomeningocele

General Features

- Meninges and spinal cord have herniated through a large vertebral defect

- Distended meningeal sac is filled with CSF and is covered by a thin membrane or skin.
- Dilatation of the central canal and herniation of the posterior cord.

Clinical Features

- Associated spinal anomalies are syringomyelia, double central canal.
- Hydrocephalus – If Arnold-Chiari malformation present.
- Lesion above T12: Lesions aboveT12 thoracic have higher incidence of spinal cord malformations. These are more common in females in comparison to the males.

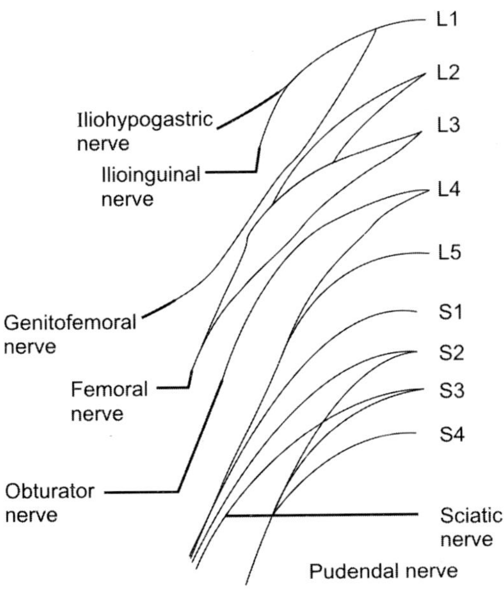

Fig. 5.3: The lumbosacral plexus

These include atresia of cerebral aqueduct, Arnold-Chiari malformation of medulla, etc. One important point to note is that where upper limbs are involved in myelomeningocele at thoracic level; this may be due to hydromyelia above externally obvious lesion of the meningomyelcele in the thoracic region.

Meningocele

General Features

- A variant of spinal bifida cystica.
- Vertebral defect combined with cystic lesion of the back.
- The defect is usually at the lumbosacral level (Fig. 5.3).
- Narrow central canal connects the cyst with vertebral canal.
- The dura and arachnoid have herniated through the vertebral defect.
- Meningocele could be associated with diastematomyelia or tethered cord.

Clinical Features

- Loss of bladder, bowel and sexual function.
- Sensory loss in the trunk and lower limbs.
- Wasting weakness of the muscles below the knee.
- Loss of ankle and knee jerks.

Spina Bifida Occulta

It is a closed defect of the embryonic neural tube that undergoes secondary canalization.

Clinical Features

- Anomalies of the anorectal and urogenital system.
- Defects are lowin lumbar and sacral region.

- Associated with teratoma, lipoma, pescavus, neurogenic bladder wasting and sensory loss in affected roots.

Syringomyelia

- The syrinx may originate at the base of the posterior horn and extend in central gray and anterior commissure.
- Lower cervical cord is the most common location although lumbar syrinx does occur.

Clinical Features

- Loss of pain and temperature at the segmental level.
- Normal sensation above and below the lesion.
- Light touch, vibration, and position sensibility are spared.
- Wasting of the muscles innervated by specifically involved anterior horns cells.
- Claw hand (thenar and hypothenar eminences involved).
- Horner's sign.
- Late bladder and bowel involvement.
- Loss of reflexes at the involved level.
- Extensor plantars and other pyramidal tract involvement signs.
- Pain may be severe, and may be of burning quality.
- Syringobulbia with cranial nerve palsies and even respiratory involvement occasionally occurs. Scoliosis of thoracic spine is seen.
- Charcot's joint of hips, shoulder occur due to loss of pain and propioception from repeated trauma.
- Autonomic features are commonly seen as diffuse swelling and subcutaneous edema, sweating.

Lumbar Syrinx

- Atrophy of proximal and distal leg muscles.
- Dissociated sensory loss in lumbar and sacral dermatomes.
- Loss of deep tendon reflexes.
- Babinski's sign is present.
- Loss of bladder and bowel function.

Tethered Cord

General Features

- Fibrous filum terminale attaches to the sacrum.
- Cord is pulled down.
- Conus medullaris is below L1.

Clinical Features

- Manifests usually in middle age.
- Pescavus is present.
- Lower limb shows asymmetrical weakness.
- Hyperactive reflexes.
- Lipoma of the sacral cord is present.

Chiari Malformation

Chiari I

General Features

- Cerebellar tonsillar herniation
- Cerebellar tonsils are atrophic and are attached to fibrous adhesions at back of the medulla.
- Often associated with late onset hydrocephalus and cerebellar ataxia.

- 50% of patients have syringomyelia.
- It is also associated with 90% of idiopathic syringomyelic patients and also with other craniocervical anomalies including platybasia, basilar invagination, craniosynostosis, Klippel-Feil anomaly, etc.

Clinical Features

- Cervical syrinx: Severe headache spreading up from C2 region to the top of the head.
- Ataxia of upper and lower extremities.
- Ataxia of gait.
- Downbeat nystagmus.

Neurogenic Cysts

- Occur in ventral thoracic cord.
- Early developmental defect.
- Signs of spinal cord compression with weakness, spasticity and bladder dysfunction.

Tethered Cord

General Features

- Fibrous filum terminale attaches to the sacrum.
- Cord is pulled down.
- It is important to note that the conus medullaris is below L1.

Clinical Features

- Late presentation often past middle age
- May start with leg weakness
- Asymmetric pescavus

- Bladder dysfunction
- Hyperactive reflexes.
- Often associated with lipoma.

Vertebral Column – Bony Disease

General Features

- These diseases may be congenital or acquired.
- It could be associated with atlantoaxial dislocation.
- The atlas has a ring like structure but no vertebral body.
- Synovial articulation occur with occipital condyles of the skull and caudally with odontoid process.
- The odontoid has three ligaments: Posterior cruciate and two lateral ligaments.
- In adults, during flexion the atlas should not move > 3 mm from the axis. In children the separation is 5 mm.
- The tip of the odontoid process should not extend rostrally more than 3 mm above the line from hard palate to the inner table of the skull at the foramen magnum (Chamberlain's line).
- Clinical features are those of paraparesis or quadriparesis and usually are preceded by cervical trauma for many years.

Occipitalization of the Atlas

There is fusion of atlas and foramen magnum.

Clinical Features

- Spastic quadriparesis
- Ataxia legs > arms
- Basilar invagination
- The odontoid process is > 3 mm above Chamberlain's line.

- The cervical spinal cord is compressed.
- Paresthesiae of hands and feet.
- Lhermitte's sign with neck flexion.
- Signs of medullary compression with cardiac arrhythmias, respiratory arrest, or sudden death.
- Short neck with decreased range of motion in all planes
- Rarely papilledema
- CSF proteins are increased.

Platybasia

General Features

- Flattening of the base of the skull.
- The normal angle between the planum sphenoidal and the clivus is 135 degrees. If this angle is increased above 135 degrees, there is platybasia.
- It may be associated with atlantoaxial dislocation, stenosis of the foramen magnum, or/and partial or complete fusion of atlas and occiput.
- Distortion of the pons, medulla, cerebellum, vertebral artery obstruction on head turning.

Clinical Features

- Vertigo.
- Drop attacks due to occlusion of vertebral artery.
- There may be lower cranial nerves, particularly glossopharyngeal and vagus nerve involvement, giving rise to swallowing difficulties and hoarseness of voice.
- Spastic paraparesis and quadriparesis.
- Ataxia arms > legs.
- The acquired defect may be due to Paget's disease, rickets, rheumatoid arthritis, etc.

TUMORS OF THE SPINAL CORD

Patterns of involvement of the spinal cord could be following:

- Epidural
- Intraparenchymal – Intramedullary
- Intradural – Extramedullary: Intradural extramedullary tumors are usually benign and could be:
  - Meningioma
  - Neurofibroma

Other tumors, which are benign, include the following:

- Schawnoma
- Ganglioneuroma
- Hemangioma
- Dermoid
- Teratoma.

Meningioma

General Features

- Arises from arachnoid cells
- Greater than 90% of meningiomas are intradural
- Peak incidence occurs between 40-70 years
- 80% of the cases occur in women
- Pain is followed by paraparesis, sensory loss and a neurogenic bladder.
- Recurrence rate is rare.

Diagnosis

Imaging on MRI shows the following features:

- Homogeneous enhancement.
- Isodense to spinal cord in T1-T2 weighted images.

Neurofibroma

General Features

- It comprises of the mixture of Schwann cell, fibroblastic and collagen fibers that grow through the nerve. They occur throughout the neuraxis.
- The condition occurs equally in men and women.
- Average age of onset is 45 years.
- 2/3 cases are intradural, while 1/3 cases are intradural + extradural (dumbbell shaped neurofibroma).

Clinical Features

- Radiculopathy – painful
- Skin stigmata: Café au lait spots
- Gradual spinal cord compression
- Weakness + spasticity below the level of the lesion.
- Babinski's sign is present
- Dropped sensory level
- Bladder involvement may be present.

Investigations

- Meniscus sign on myelography
- Scalloped vertebral body.

Epidural Tumors

General Features

- Majority are metastatic
- Commonest malignancies are breast, prostate, lymphoma, and melanoma of GI tract

- Others include, multiple myeloma, chordoma, etc.
- They reach epidural space by hematogenous spread
- Majority of cases, i.e. 70% are thoracic; 20% are lumbosacral; 10% cervical
- Melanoma may metastasize to digits, heart surface and intestinal wall in addition to the epidural space.

Clinical Features

- Boring pain in the back, which worsens in recumbent posture and is exacerbated at night.
- Gait ataxia precedes weakness due to involvement of spinocerebellar tract, both dorsal and ventral.
- Weakness may precede other sensory symptoms
- Bladder involvement is late.

Diagnosis

Laboratory evaluation:
- Malignant cells in the CSF
- Glucose levels 30-40 mg%
- Protein levels 80 to 150 mg%

Imaging:
- Pedicle involvement
- Erosion of the endplates and central vertebral body lesions, noted on plain film suggest metastatic disease.

MRI:
- Pathologic fractures
- Osteoblastic bone changes
- Multiple areas of T1 weighted low density areas in the vertebra.

Intraparenchymal Tumors

- Astrocytoma
- Ependymoma
- Intramedullary metastasis
- Medulloblastoma.

DEMYELINATING SPINAL CORD DISEASE

Multiple Sclerosis

Similar to Europe and America, in Asia too incidence and prevalence of multiple sclerosis is rising. With newer imaging techniques, better diagnostic criteria have been enunciated to increase epidemiological yield of multiple sclerosis. Unfortunately visual evoked response and CSF immunoglobulins did not prove to be fully useful for diagnosing this disease.

There occurs great deal of similarity in presentation of multiple sclerosis in its spinal form with spinal cord compression. Prior to the advent of the newer imaging modalities, myelography was the only definitive method of excluding compression. Also, in many patients with demyelinating plaques in the spinal cord, the condition worsened after myelography. There were too occasions when multiple sclerosis diagnosis being made by clinical methods alone, left many patients with progressive spinal cord affectation. In these cases, the neurologist had made the diagnosis of multiple sclerosis without recourse to myelography as the neurosurgeon did not think that the myelography was necessary. By the time, myelography was done on such patients, there had already been much damage done to the spinal cord and it became difficult for the neurosurgeon to salvage whatever that was left of the viable cord by decompressive measures such as removal of benign tumors like neurofibroma or meningioma or neurogenic cyst.

Clinical presentation of multiple sclerosis: Spinal cord is affected in majority of cases of multiple sclerosis. There are principally three patterns of clinical presentations:

- Neuropathic type
- Subacute cord compression
- Acute transverse myelitis

Associated neurological findings include bilateral cerebellar ataxia, loss of abdominal reflexes, internuclear ophthalmoplegia and afferent pupillary defects.

Neuropathic Type

Sensory symptoms predominate: These may be in the form of numbness and tingling which may be exactly like those seen in peripheral neuropathy and involve distal arms and legs. Lhermitte's phenomenon, manifested by electric shock like sensation passing down the center of the back or legs when the neck is flexed, is often present. This may involve all four limbs or only arms, lower limbs or the back.

It is not pathognomic sign of multiple sclerosis, but is also seen in cervical myelopathy due to spondylosis or cervical tumors. The clue which helps to point to spinal cord lesion rather than peripheral lesion are the reflexes which are brisk to exaggerated and the plantars are extensors.

The abdominal reflexes are usually absent and pyramidal signs are present. This presentation is seen in younger age group 18 to 30 years and there is very little progression to motor involvement. The prognosis is good and remissions do occur.

Subacute Cord Compression

It may present as progressive spastic paraparesis. MRI is the only definitive means of excluding compression such as due to cervical myelopathy or that which is secondary to cervical spondylosis in the older age group.

Acute Transverse Myelitis

It is the most serious presentation of spinal cord demyelination.

Clinical Features

- Clinical features are that of spinal cord transection.
- It may occur instantaneously or over 2-3 days.
- Thoracic cord is the commonest site of affectation.
- Acutely it manifests as flaccid paralysis of the lower limbs with urinary retention.
- Clear cut sensory level.

Devic's Disease

Acute transverse myelitis with bilateral optic neuritis is known as Devic's disease. Onset may be simultaneous or can occur a separate episodes months apart. It is common presentation of MS in Asian patients.

SPINAL CORD VASCULAR DISEASES

These are:

1. Arterial
2. Venous

Arterial: Commonest pathogenic mechanism is atherosclerosis of vertebral artery and orifice of anterior spinal artery.

Other causes include:
- Syphilis
- Sarcoid
- Vasculitis due to SLE, collagen vascular disease.
- Emboli from the heart due to atrial fibrillation, or subacute bacterial endocarditis.
- Takayasu's disease.

It can present as medullary syndrome with high anterior spinal artery occlusion.

Clinical Features

- Ipsilateral XII nerve paralysis.
- Contralateral weakness of arms and legs.
- Anterior spinal artery occlusion at lower level.
- When 2/3 of ventral spinal cord is involved, there is weakness of extremities below the lesion.
- Loss of pain and temperature sensation below the lesion.
- Dorsal column – sensation intact.

Ischemia of Spinal Cord

The blood supply of spinal cord is such that there are certain watershed areas in the spinal cord which are susceptible to damage as the perfusion pressure falls below critical level. This may occur in isolation, affecting spinal cord segment at T4-T6 level and the most damage is done to corticospinal tract. Clinical settings in which this may occur include:
- Renal arteriogram.
- Clamping of the aorta during surgical procedures.
- Dissection of the aorta.
- Emboli from the heart.
- Atherosclerosis.

Often the spinal cord is infarcted in association with cerebral anoxic insult following cardiac arrest, carbon monoxide poisoning or vertebral artery atherosclerotic occlusion.

Venous Infarction of the Cord

The venous infarction of the spinal cord is not different from arterial infarction. The clue to diagnosis of venous infarction is its association with hemorrhage. This may be in epidural space, intradural or extramedullary space and often intraparenchymatous. The latter is designated as hematomyelia and occurs under specific conditions which are mentioned in later section.

Principally common underlying medical conditions which predispose to venous infarction are:

a. Thrombophlebitis of pelvic veins.
b. Polycythemia vera.
c. Coagulopathy due to factor C deficiency, antiphospholipid syndrome, lupus anticoagulant, etc.
d. Oral contraceptive pills.
e. Pregnancy.
f. Dehydration.
g. Disseminated intravascular coagulation.
h. Antiphospholipid syndrome.
i. Factor V leiden mutation with protein C resistance.
j. Malignancy of breast, and pancreas is most common setting.

Primary Hemorrhagic Diseases of Spinal Cord

Primary hemorrhagic diseases of spinal cord usually occur in the following categories:

1. Spinal angioma

2. Spinal arteriovenous malformation
3. Telangiectasiae.

Clinical Features

Progressive paraparesis or radiculopathy.

Transverse Myelitis – Acute Onset

Clinical Features

- Severe back pain
- Symptoms may worsen with exercise and mimic MS.

Diagnosis

Imaging evaluation:
- Increased T2 weighted signal with edema in the cord by MRI imaging.
- Digital spinal angiography is the investigation of choice and can complement magnetic resonance angiography.

Spinal Cord Subarachnoid Hemorrhage

Etiology

Common causes are:
- Rupture of arteriovenous malformations
- Blood dyscrasias
- Drug sensitivity

Clinical Features

- Acute onset.
- Severe back pain usually at the site of hemorrhage, but uniformly spreading over the spinal segments.

- Pain, sometimes radiates to the shoulder between the interscapular region or to the legs.
- Signs of meningeal irritation are common. These include intense photophobia, neck stiffness, Kernig's sign positive.
- With diffusion of blood in the region of the foramen magnum, unconsciousness may prevail.
- In association with cranial nerve palsies, papilledema may be seen.

Diagnosis

Laboratory evaluation:

- MRI may show ruptured AVM.
- *CSF:* Markedly raised RBC count in a hemorrhagic CSF.
- Spinal hemorrhage may also occur in epidural space and present more often as progressive paraparesis or rarely as Brown-Séquard's syndrome.
- Cauda-Equina syndrome.
- MRI is usually of diagnostic value demonstrating signal intensity isodense to that of spinal cord.
- Spinal epidural hemorrhage usually occurs following trivial trauma or exertion in children.

Spastic Paraplegias

Spastic paraplegias can be of two types: Hereditary and Acquired.

Hereditary Spastic Paraplegias

- Hereditary spastic paraplegias has been more recently described to be a genetically heterogenous disorder.
- Both recessive and dominant inheritance has been described.

- 18 genetic loci have been identified of which 10 are autosomal dominant; 3 X-linked; and 5 autosomal recessive.
- In the pure form of hereditary spastic paraplegias, both corticospinal and dorsal column tracts are involved.
- Complicated HSP have additional neurological deficits, which include optic neuritis macular and cerebellar degeneration, seizures, cognitive dysfunction, extrapyramidal signs, ichthyosis, etc.

Autosomal Dominant Hereditary Spastic Paraplegias

Type I age ‹ 35 years
Type II age › 35 years.

Clinical Features

AD type I:
- Motor delay
- Abnormal gait
- Hyperreflexia
- Distal sensory loss
- Spasticity paraparesis
- Abnormal gait.

AD Type II:
- Weakness 47%
- Areflexia 20%
- Hyperreflexia
- Bladder disorder › 50%
- No bowel disturbance.

Autosomal recessive:
- Chromosome 8 Q
- Onset is in 1st decade

- Spastic gait
- Weakness of legs
- Pescavus.

AR complicated form:
- Associated with dysphagia and dysarthria
- Optic atrophy
- Axonal neuropathy
- Mitochondrial defects on muscle biopsy.

X-linked recessive HSP:
- Corpus callosum is thin
- Mental retardation
- Hydrocephalus
- Spastic paraparesis.

Complicated form:
- Hydrocephalus
- Aphasia.

Pure form:
- Onset during 2nd decade
- Spastic gait
- Spasticity
- No weakness
- No pescavus.

Machado-Joseph Disease

- Chromosome 14
- Spastic paraparesis
- Ataxia
- External ophthalmoplegia.

Adrenoleukodystrophy

- Onset after 2nd decade
- Progressive spastic paraparesis
- Sensory loss in legs
- Sphincter disturbance
- Hypogonadism.

Metachromatic Leukodystrophy

- Late infantile onset 6 months to 2 years
- Juvenile onset 3 to 16 years
- Behavioral abnormalities.

Spastic Paraparesis

Pathology

- Metachromatic inclusions within Schwann cell and macrophages.
- Segmental peripheral nerve demyelination.

Acquired Spastic Paraplegias

These include tropical spastic paraparesis and HTLV-1 myelitis.

At the beginning of 1980, most cases of endemic TSP were considered to be due to an undetermined cause; nevertheless similar picture was attributed to nutritional deficiencies, including neurotoxins such as lathyrus sativus as well as various bacterial and parasitic infections. With the discovery and isolation of first human reterovirus from a patient with cutaneous T-cell lymphoma and subsequent demonstration that the human T-lymphotropic virus type I (HTLV-1) as the causal agent of adult T-cell leukemia, it became clear that HTLV-I is also a neurotropic virus. This virus has been linked to tropical spastic paraparesis.

Clinical Features

- The basic clinical feature in different regions of the world is uniform.
- In 60% of cases onset is gradual, but acute onset similar to spinal stroke or transverse myelitis does occur in few percentage of cases.
- Clinical features including asymmetrical leg weakness, back pain, numbness, stiffness bladder and bowel disorder and sexual impotence are common.
- Signs are those of pyramidal tract involvement.
- There is minimal posterior column involvement.
- Proximal lower limb muscle weakness may be present.

Diagnosis

- Serum protein electrophoresis shows that 30% of the patients have elevations of IgG and IgA.
- CSF is normal.
- Trepenoma pallidum antibodies have been demonstrated in 60% of patients.
- Blood brain barrier is intact and increased intrathecal synthesis of IgG antibodies against HTLV-1 is demonstrated by specific IgG index or presence of oligoclonal bands on isoelectric focusing.

Radiation Myelopathy

Spinal cord may be subjected to radiation damage at cervical, thoracic, and lumbar regions. This usually results due to secondary damage to spinal cord following radiotherapy treatment for carcinoma of the bronchus, oesophagus and Hodgkin's disease.

Onset usually occurs at 9-18 months following treatment, but can also occur after 1-2 months or as late as 24 months after treatment.

Clinical Features

Predominant spinothalamic tract involvement may produce sensory symptoms, coldness, numbness, stiffness and weakness of legs. Motor symptoms and signs are less prominent. This is the first clue which differentiates radiation myelopathy from spinal cord compression.

A variant of this myelopathy has been recently described in long-term survivors of radiation to the para-aortic lymph nodes in the treatment of malignancy of testis.

It exactly mimics motor neuron disease in clinical presentation and produces symptoms like wasting, weakness, and fasciculation of leg muscles. All muscles supplied by lumbar, sacral roots are involved.

SPINAL CORD METABOLIC AND NUTRITIONAL

Subacute Combined Degeneration of the Spinal Cord

This disease of the spinal cord follows B_{12} deficiency. In earlier years it was a frequent complication of pernicious anemia. About a quarter of patients who have CNS involvement do not have hematological abnormalities. Therefore, in all cases of probable nutritional cause or spinal cord damage, serum B_{12} estimation is to be done.

Besides autoimmune cause due to lack of intrinsic factor other causes of B_{12} deficiency are following: Total gastrectomy, blindloop syndrome, infestation with tapeworm and Crohn's disease. Strict vegetarians too develop B_{12} deficiency.

Clinical Features

The clinical features are signs of peripheral nerve damage and include the following:

- Tingling, numbness of legs, and areflexia.
- Minimal evidence of corticospinal damage in the form of extensor plantar.
- Bladder disturbance in the form of retention of urine.
- Cerebral involvement is common.
- Early signs of cognitive decline.
- Early estimation of serum B_{12} is to be done to avoid irreversible damage to corticospinal tract so that substitution therapy with B_{12} can be instituted.

6 Cerebellum

ANATOMY

Cerebellum is located in the posterior cranial fossa underneath tentorium cerebelli and behind the pons and medulla oblongata. It is separated from pons and medulla by the cavity of the fourth ventricle. Its surface has numerous fissures separating narrow folia (Fig. 6.1). The cerebellum is connected to the brainstem by cerebellar peduncles.

It maintains equilibrium, muscle tone and posture. It also coordinates skillful volitional movements by timing activities of both antagonists and agonists muscles. This is achieved by receiving input from joint and muscles and then modulating motor outputs from cerebrum and brainstem. It is manifested in form of motor disturbances, unsteady gait, hypotonia and loss of coordination.

The two cerebellar hemispheres are united by vermis, which has two parts: Superior and inferior vermis.

Notches of cerebellum viz anterior cerebellar notch and posterior cerebellar notch lodge pons, medulla and falx cerebelli respectively.

The three parts of cerebellum are:

1. Archicerebellum
2. Paleocerebellum
3. Neocerebellum.

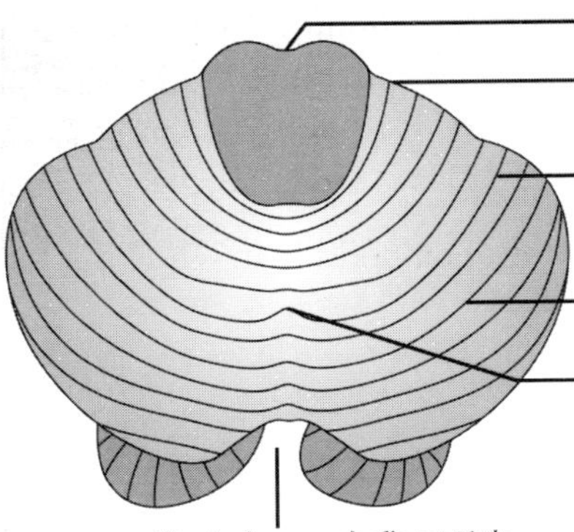

Fig. 6.1: Superior view of the cerebellum

Each part has distinct functions:

- Archicerebellum chiefly is concerned with maintenance of equilibrium, tone and posture of trunk muscles.
- Paleocerebellum has spinocerebellar connections and is concerned with tone, posture and crude movements of the limbs.
- Neocerebellum is concerned with skilled voluntary movements.

Internal Structure of the Cerebellum

- Outer molecular layer
- Intermediate Purkinje cell layer
- Inner granular layer.

There are five distinct types of neurons in the cerebellum:

1. Purkinje cell
2. Granule cells
3. Stellate cells

4. Basket cells
5. Golgi cell.

Intracerebellar Nuclei

They are masses of gray matter embedded in white matter of cerebellum.

These include:

1. Dentate nucleus
2. Emboliform nucleus
3. Globose nucleus
4. Fastigial nucleus

The white matter of the cerebellum has intrinsic and efferent and afferent fibers.

- Intrinsic fibers connect each of the hemisphere and different regions of the cerebellum.
- The afferent and efferent fibers connect cerebellum.
- The afferent fibers bring input to the cerebellum from cerebral cortex, spinal cord, and vestibular apparatus.
- Efferent fibers carry output to the red nucleus, thalamus, vestibular complex, reticular formation. These afferent and efferent fibers are grouped on either side into three large bundles called cerebellar peduncles.

Blood Supply

- Superior cerebellar artery supplies superior surface of the cerebellum.
- Anterior inferior cerebellar artery supplies anterior part of the inferior surface of the cerebellum.
- Superior cerebellar artery and anterior inferior cerebellar artery are branches of basilar artery.

- The posterior inferior cerebellar artery, branch of the vertebral artery supplies posterior part of the inferior surface of the cerebellum.

Clinical Signs of Cerebellar Disease

Ataxia

Gait ataxia: Staggering gait gross.

Minimal ataxia: Elicited by asking the patient to walk in a straight line – Tandem walking.

Truncal ataxia is a feature of midline cerebellar lesion. Patient is unable to sit or stand without support may fall backwards. It is a sign of midline cerebellar tumor, cyst. or degeneration. The commonest tumors are medulloblastoma and metastasis. Sometimes encephalitis also gives rise to truncal ataxia.

Limb Ataxia

Limb ataxia is tested by finger nose finger test. This test assesses the patient's ability to touch the tip of the nose with his index finger and then with examiners index finger and noting for ataxia of the index finger. It is also tested in the legs the heel/knee/shin.

This test is performed by placing the tip of the heel on the tibial tubercle of the other leg and then run down the heel on the front of the shin. Then the heel is lifted and again placed on the tibial tubercle. If positive on one side, it indicates disease of the cerebellum on the same side as ataxia.

Rebound Phenomenon

Rebound phenomenon is tested by noting the patients' inability to check movements of their outstretched hands. The patient keeps his hands outstretched then the examiner presses down on the hand and suddenly releases the pressure. In normal individual, on releasing the pressure, the out stretched hand returns back immediately to the original position. In cerebellar disease, the hand oscillates up and down, few motions before returning back to the original position. In this process the hand may completely fly up out of control before normal position is assumed.

Rapid Alternating Movements: Dysdiadochokinesis

Dysdiadochokinesis refers to the impairment of the patients ability to perform rapidly alternating movements. This is tested by asking the patient to tap the back of one hand with palm of the other. In abnormal situation the movements are slow and dysonchronised.

Tremors

Intention tremors may appear on performing actions such as on finger to nose test.

Truncal Tremor

Truncal tremors refer to constant backward and forward jerking of the body.

Tone

Reduced tone: In cerebellar diseases, the tone is often reduced.

Reflexes

Reflexes, although brisk, there may sometimes be a slow, to an from movement on tapping the tendon of the affected limb.

This is what is known as pendular jerk and is best demonstrated at the knees. The knee jerk reflex is mediated by the L3 and L4 nerve roots, mainly L4. Insult to the cerebellum may lead to pendular reflexes, which are not brisk but involve less damping of the limb movement than is usually observed when a deep tendon reflex is elicited. Patients with cerebellar injury may have a knee jerk that swings forwards and backwards several times. On the other hand, a normal or brisk knee jerk would have little more than one swing forward and one back. Pendular reflexes are best observed when the patient's lower legs are allowed to hang and swing freely off the end of an examining table.

Nystagmus

Variety of nystagmus are seen in cerebellar disease. These are vertical nystagmus, horizontal gaze nystagmus, and rotatory nystagmus.

Dysarthria

The speech disturbances could be in the form of scanning speech, slurred speech, and explosive type of speech with pauses.

Other Symptoms

Headache: Similar to the patients with raised intracranial tension, vomiting of projectile type may occur on sitting up or lying down.

DISEASES OF CEREBELLUM

Diseases of the cerebellum could be of various types as follows:

1. Vascular
2. Degenerative

3. Infective
4. Toxic
5. Tumors
6. Congenial.

Vascular

Vascular disease of the cerebellum could be due to the infarction of different cerebellar vessels as described below:

Posterior Inferior Cerebellar Artery Infarction

Clinical Features

- Nausea
- Vomiting
- Ataxia
- Vestibular signs: Vertigo, dysmetria, and dysarthria.
- Sensory loss to pain and temperature on the ipsilateral face and contralateral body.

Anterior Inferior Cerebellar Artery Infarction

Clinical Features

- Sudden hearing loss
- Lower motor facial weakness
- Ataxia of the arms, greater than legs.

Superior Cerebellar Artery Infarction

- Ataxia of all extremities.
- Dysarthria
- Thalamic sensory loss

- Midbrain, and parietal lobe signs and symptoms
- Clumsy hand
- Dysarthria syndrome.

AUTOSOMAL RECESSIVE HEREDITARY ATAXIAS

General Features

- Autosomal recessive mode of inheritence
- Childhood onset
- Consanguinity higher than general population.

Friedreich's Ataxia

- Prevalence of 2 per 100,000 people
- Chromosome 9Q13 FRDA gene is involved
- There may be hypertrophic cardiomyopathy or diabetes mellitus.

Clinical Features

- Onset occurs at less than 25 years of age
- Progressive gait ataxia
- Scoliosis
- Pescavus
- Extensor plantars
- Dysphagia
- Optic atrophy
- 8th nerve deafness.

Diagnosis

MRI

- Cerebellar atrophy
- Atrophy of upper cervical cord.

EMG

- Decrease of sensory nerve action potential (SNAP)
- Central conduction defects.

Ataxia Telangiectasis

- Autosomsal recessive inheritance
- 1:400,000 births in USA
- Common in ethnic groups with consangunity.

Clinical Features

- Ataxia by age two
- Wheelchair bound by 12 years of age.
- Oculomotor apraxia
- Dysarthria
- Short stature
- Mental retardation
- Choreoathetosis
- Lymphoid cancer occurs in 1/3 of patients.

Laboratory evaluation:

- Deficiency of IGA, IGE and Ig2
- Elevated albumin/Globulin ratio
- Decreased ATM proteins.

Ataxia with Vitamin E Deficiency

Clinical Features

- Progressive ataxia
- Propioceptive loss
- Areflexia
- Retinal disease
- Rarely, cardiomyopathy may occur.

Diagnosis

Laboratory:
Decreased alpha tocopherol levels.

Ramsay Hunt Syndrome

- Autosomal recessive inheritance.
- Progressive cerebellar ataxia
- Myoclonus
- Dementia
- Seizures
- *Baltic myoclonus* (Unverricht-Lundborg syndrome)
- Chromosone 21Q gene cystatin, β stimulus sensitive myoclonus
- Seizures
- Ataxia
- Pyramidal tract dysfunction.

Autosomal Dominant Ataxia

Clinical Features

- Ophthalmoplegia.
- Optic atrophy
- Peripheral neuropathy
- Pyramidal and extrapyramidal signs.
- Genetic heterogeneity
- Onset from 3rd to 5th decades.

Congenital Defects of Cerebellum

General Characteristics

May occur as a consequence of neuronal migration from external granular layer.

It occurs *in utero* at 32 weeks of gestation and develops up to one year.

There may be other factors such as toxins affecting cerebellum; some of these include drugs, chemicals, hypoxia, viral infections, etc.

Clinical Features

- Hypoplasia or aplasia of the vermis with intact lateral ventricles associated with midline defects such as agenesis of corpus callosum.
- Abnormal eye movements
- Ataxia
- Mental retardation.

DANDY-WALKER SYNDROME

General Features

- Large posterior one-half of the fourth ventricle along with atresia of foramen of Magendie.
- Pachygyria of cerebral cortex
- Hydrocephalus.

Clinical Features

- Mental retardation
- Spastic diplegia.

ARNOLD-CHIARI MALFORMATION

- Chiari I
- Chiari II
- Chiari III
- Chiari IV

Clinical Features

- Sudden ataxia
- Shallow posterior fossa
- Low hairline
- Increased reflexes.

METABOLIC ATAXIAS

General Features

- Onset in infancy or childhood
- Urea cycle defects
- Amino acidurias
- Autosomal recessive inheritance.

Hartnup Disease

- Autosomal recessive inheritance.

Clinical Features

- Ataxia
- Tremor
- Chorea
- Mental retardation.

TUMORS OF THE CEREBELLUM

General Features

- In general tumors of the cerebellum are age specific.
- Children and adults may present with cerebellar symptoms and signs due to ependymoma.
- Hydrocephalus, and papilledema are prominent features.
- Medulloblastoma may also present with similar features.

- Solid and cystic astrocytomas may be from cerebellar hemisphere or vermis. These tumors may distort IVth ventricle and press on pons and medulla.
- Headache, vomiting and bilateral sixth nerve palsy may occur.
- Rare tumors are oligodendroglioma, which is to a large part benign, but may exhibit malignant change.
- Hemangioblastoma are vascular tumors and can be picked up on MRI.
- Cerebellopontine angle tumors are; (I) Schwannoma (II) Meningioma (III) Epidermoid.
- Metastatic lesions are common and are usually from lungs, breast and GI tract primaries.
- Lymphomas may be seen in HIV positive patients.

Metabolic Disorders

Metabolic disorders giving rise to cerebellar syndromes are:
- Hyperosmolar syndromes due to dehydration, diabetes, causing hypernatremia may present with ataxia and myoclonus.
- Hyponatremia correction at a rapid pace causes positive myelinolysis – Due to destruction of pontine fibers constituting cerebellar peduncles.

Autoimmune Diseases

Autoimmune disorders like chronic inflammatory demyelinating peripheral neuropathy and Guillain-Barré syndrome also present with cerebellar features particularly CIDP, which may be detected on MRI.

Systemic lupus erythematosus occasionally gives rise to acute cerebellar syndrome due to vasculitis.

Demyelinating Diseases

Multiple sclerosis:

- Cerebellar signs are common.
- Frontal lobe mental changes are seen associated with internuclear ophthalmoplegia, optic neuritis, and spasticity.

Acute disseminated encephalomyelitis: Frequently evolves into multiple sclerosis.

Postviral encephalitis: May show cerebellar signs and on MRI periventricular lucency is seen.

7 The Extrapyramidal System

The basal ganglia forms essential constituent of the extrapyramidal system.

Basal ganglia includes (Fig. 7.1)

- Corpus callosum
- Claustrum
- Amygdaloid body.

Functionally it also includes substantia nigra, red nucleus, and subthalamus. They are important in organizing and coordinating motor movements and posture. Corpus callosum situated lateral to the thalamus is divided into the caudate nucleus and the lentiform nucleus by internal capsule.

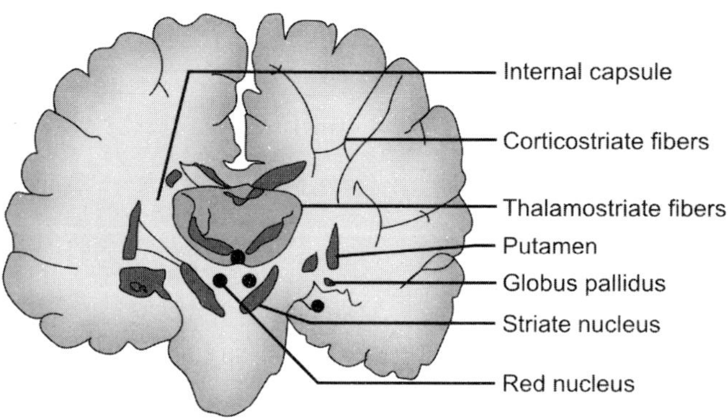

Fig. 7.1: The basal ganglia and thalamus

Lentiform nucleus consists of putamen and globus pallidus.

CONNECTIONS OF THE CORPUS STRIATUM

The connections of the corpus striatum are summarized in Figure 7.2.

Afferent Connections

The striatum receives afferents chiefly from cerebral cortex, thalamus and substantia nigra. These include corticostriate, thalamostriate and nigrostriate fibers.

The nigrostriate fibers carry dopamine synthesized by nerve cells of substantia nigra to the striatum.

Efferent Connections

Most of the output of the striatum goes to the globus pallidus and some to substantia nigra. From the globus pallidus the outflow is to the thalamus.

Functions of the Corpus Callosum

- Controls associated movements of the limbs like swinging of the arms during walking.
- Smoothens voluntary activity of the body.
- *Claustrum:* It is situated between putamen and insula. Its functions are not known.
- *Amygdaloid body:* It is situated deep to the uncus and is an almond shaped mass of the grey matter in the temporal lobe.
- *Substantia nigra:* It is situated between tegmentum and crus cerebri. It is made up of deeply pigmented nerve cells which

contain melanin and iron. These cells synthesize dopamine which is carried to the striatum by the axons.

- *Subthalamus (subthalamic nucleus):* It is located caudal to the lateral half of the thalamus and inferiomedial to the globus pallidus.
- The activity of the basal ganglia is initiated by information received from the cerebral cortex, the thalamus and the brainstem. The outflow from the basal ganglia is channeled through the globus pallidus, which then influences the activities of the motor areas of the cerebral cortex.
- Principal functions of basal ganglia are concerned with planning and programming of voluntary movement. Regulate muscle tone control reflex muscular activity.

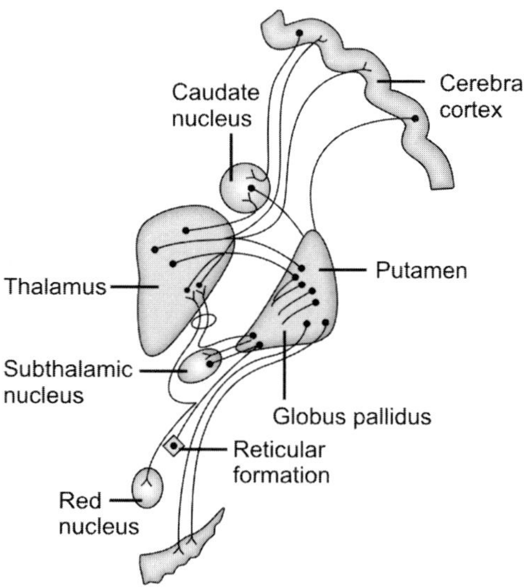

Fig. 7.2: Corpus striatum afferent and efferent connections

Clinical Features of Diseases of Extrapyramidal System

Tremor

Important feature is that rhythm is constant, amplitude may vary.
There are three clinically distinct forms of tremors.

Rest tremor: Rest tremors are seen in Parkinson's disease, important feature being that the tremor diminishes on performing action; holding the hand straight out diminishes the tremor. In Parkinson's disease the tremor is best observed when the patient is distracted.

Action tremor (Intention tremor): This is seen in cerebellar diseases, demonstrated on finger nose finger test. The differentiating point between cerebellar tremor (Rubrodentate) and Parkinsonian tremor is that cerebellar tremor accentuates at the end of volitional movement such as finger nose finger test, while Parkinsonian tremors stop on movement. In case of action tremors, if the action continues, the tremor remains constant throughout the range.

Red nucleus tremor: It is a violent tremor as manifested in multiple sclerosis or midbrain vascular disease. Often it is accompanied by truncal and nuchal ataxia and inarticulate speech. The lesion causing this tremor can be anywhere along the dentatorubro thalamic tract and is not specifically confined to the red nucleus itself.

Hemiballismus

It is characterized by violent wild flinging movements of the upper limb when the patient tries to move from resting position.

Thus, abnormal movement is seen following infarction or hemorrhage resulting in damage to subthalamic nucleus. This rare condition may respond to surgical intervention - stereotactic surgery involving subthalamic nucleus. Chlorpromazine 25 mg intravenously produces immediate relief and subsequently oral chlorpromazine helps in controlling the movements.

Chorea

Choreiform movements are sudden, rapid, involuntary, jerky, purposeless movements which interrupt patient's normal activity.

Athetosis

These are slow writhing sinuous movements of the arms and legs, best demonstrated by holding the arms outstretched when the arm becomes extended and internally rotated. The foot is inverted and plantar flexed. Dystonic movements often accompany these athetoid movements.

Dystonia

These are slow prolonged contractions of the trunk muscles. There is hyperextension of the head, and twisting, and lateral flexion of the spine.

Dystonia may include the following movements:

a. Spasmodic torticollis - Head is pulled to one side.
b. Writer's cramp
c. Blepharospasm
d. Various facial distortions like tongue protrusions, contractions of platysma, and other facial muscles.

Myoclonus

This includes sudden brief shock like jerks involving a group of muscles, or a single muscle. Sometimes the force of the jerks may throw the patient on the ground.

Tics

They may take the form of movements such as sniffing, grunting, snorting, pouting, clearing the throat, shoulder shrugging, grimacings, winking, etc.

The most common condition associated with tics, described in form of a syndrome is known as Gilles de la Tourette's syndrome. In this disorder the abnormal movements are accompanied by foul utterances. It responds to phenothiazines. It normally shows an autosomal dominant type of inheritance pattern and is commonly seen in young boys.

Other clinical signs, which are more specific to particular diseases such as rigidity, bradykinesia, reflex changes are discussed in detail under section of diseases affecting extrapyramidal system.

DISEASES AFFECTING THE EXTRAPYRAMIDAL SYSTEM

Parkinson's Disease

- Incidence 4/1000 over the age of 40
- Equally affects both sexes
- Prevalence rate varies worldwide.

Risk factors:

- Rural living
- Age (commonly occurs above the age of 40)

- Exposure to well water
- Industrial exposure or exposure to chemicals like MPTP (1-methyl-4-phenyl-1,2,3,6-tetrahydropyridine), manganese, etc.
- Reduced risk with smoking
- Family history of essential tremor
- History of minor head trauma.

Genetic Aspects

- Mendelian PD genes
- Park 1 to Park II, for instance park I Chromosome 4Q 21 alphasynuclein; gene park II Chromosome 6Q 25.2-27 parkin AR; park I (Alphasynuclein).

Clinical Features

- Mean age of onset 46 years
- Cortical dementia 20%.
- Tremor at rest.
- Park 2 gene is parkin AR 6Q 25.
- Onset may be at age, less than 21 years. This may be the presentation in the recently described syndrome of young Parkinsonian disease, which occurs below the age of 21 years.
- Slow progression
- Symmetrical presentation.
- Excellent response to levodopa.
- Earlier onset of psychiatric features.

Familial Parkinsonism

Parkinsonism may be a feature of many disorders like:
- Wilson's disease
- Hallervorden - Spatz disease

- Tau associated disease
- Frontotemporal dementia
- Parkinsonism.

Genetics

- Autosomal dominant inheritance
- Chromosome on 17.

Clinical Variants

- Rigidity, bradykinesia loss of postural reflexes, personality disorders.
- Pathology: Atrophy and spongiform degeneration in the frontotemporal cortex.
- Neuronal loss and gliosis in the amygdala
- No lewy bodies.

Pallido Ponto Nigral Degeneration

- Dementia
- Dystonia
- Increased reflexes
- No amyotrophy.

Trinucleotide – Repeat Disorders

- Huntington's disease
- Spinocerebellar disease: Associated with cerebellar ataxia
- Cognitive dysfunction, chorea, anterior horn cell disease.
- Autosomal dominant spinocerebellar ataxias.
- SCA 3/Machado-Joseph disease and SCA2
- PETSCANS have demonstrated basal ganglia hypometabolism.

- SCA-2 parkinsonism symptoms are more common in Chinese and Caucasian patients.
- SCA-3 parkinsonism is more common in Afrocarribean patients
- Responsive to L-dopa.

Parkinsonism in Juvenile Variant of Huntington's Disease

- Presents in teens
- Akinetic rigid syndrome
- Seizures.

Parkinsonism Features of Wilson's Disease

- AD inheritance affecting the chromosome 13Q 14-21
- Onset at 6-40 years of age
- Psychiatric presentation neurologic or as liver disease
- Dysarthria
- Wingbeating tremors
- Dystonia
- Kayser-Fleischer ring in cornea, depression, personality changes, emotional lability with cognitive decline.

Laboratory Evaluation

- Increased urinary copper excretion (more than 100 ug/ 24 hrs),
- Low plasma ceruloplasmin levels of less than 15 ug/dl.
- MRI shows ventricular dilatation, cortical atrophy, and basal ganglia (putamen and caudate) lesions.

Parkinsonism Features of Huntington's Disease

- Chromosome 4P 16.3
- Gene is IT 15

Clinical Features

- Usual age of onset 20-50 years. Childhood onset is rare Presents with neurological and psychiatric features: Changes in personality, chorea, lurching gait, bradykinesia, and increased reflexes and clonus
- MRI may show atrophy of the caudate nucleus, and frontal lobe atrophy.

Genetics

- Autosomal dominant mode of inheritance.

Treatment

- No known treatment is available.
- Symptomatic relief may be achieved by tetrabenazine in a dose of 12.5 to 25.5 mg + TDS.
- Autosomal dominant mode of inheritance
- Lewy body positive.

Parkinsonism with atypical features:
- Autosomal dominant
- Lewy bodies present
- Late onset dementia
- Depression
- Ataxia
- Seizures.

Idiopathic Parkinsonism

General Characteristics

- Degeneration of components of the substantia pars compacta
- Lewy body formation.

Cardinal Signs

- Akinesia - bradykinesia
- Tremors at rest
- Cogwheel type of rigidity
- Autonomic dysfunction
- More than 50% patients show cognitive decline
- Bradykinesia is seen in early stage of the disease and also during off episodes at the end of effective therapy with L-dopa.
- They may experience freezing episodes especially while walking or turning or going through a doorway.

Tremors

It occurs at rest at constant speed of 4 to 6 HZ and is pathognomonic of Parkinson's disease. It occurs in the hand, involves the arm, leg may be involved.

- Responds well to L-dopa.
- Rigidity
- Contributes to stooped flexed posture of the patient
- Generalized stiffness of the body
- Loss of postural reflexes
- Results in frequent falls with hip fractures and humeral fractures.
- Patients tend to fall backwards.

Autonomic dysfunctions:

- Difficulty in initiating micturition
- Sexual dysfunction
- Postural hypotension.

Cognitive decline:

- Depression
- Decreased short-term memory
- When on dopamine therapy: Hallucinations.

Associated neurological deficits:
- Sleep disruption due to sleep apnea and REM sleep disorder.
- Decreased spontaneous blink and all subconscious movements.

Striato Nigral Degeneration

- Severe akinetic rigid syndrome
- Minimal tremor
- No response to L- dopa
- Dystonia of upper extremity
- MRI demonstrates atrophy and signal changes in the putamen.

Corticobasal Degeneration

- Degeneration of cortical areas like substantia nigra, basal ganglia, etc.
- Glial and neuronal accumulation of tau protein.

Clinical Features

- Average age 60 years
- 6 to 10 years duration
- Rigidity
- Stiffness
- Clumsiness
- Postural instability
- Progresses to dysarthria
- Dysphagia
- Supranuclear gaze palsy
- Asymmetric cortical atrophy involving frontal and parietal Lobe. Seen on neuroimaging MRI, SPECT.

Lewy Body Dementia

Hallmark is the accumulation of Lewy bodies throughout the cortex to a greater degree than Idiopathic Parkinson's disease (IPD) and aging.

Clinical Features

- Onset is in sixth to seventh decade.
- Effect on visual spatial attention and problem-solving ability are seen early.
- There may be fluctuation in cognitive abilities.
- Repeated falls.
- Syncope.
- Transient loss of consciousness.
- Transient ischemic like episodes like in IPD: Rest tremor, rigidity, bradykinesia but to a lesser degree.

Progressive Supranuclear Palsy

- Responds poorly to levodopa.
- Age of onset 64 years.
- Poor vertical saccades.
- Abnormal smooth pursuit of eye movements.
- Blepharospasms.
- Apraxia of eye opening, ptosis, decreased blinking, nystagmus, late, complete ophthalmoplegia.
- Cognitive decline, gait disturbance such as falling backward.
- Dysphagia, dysarthria.

MRI/CT Evaluation

Midbrain atrophy.

Drug Induced Parkinsonism (MPTP)

MTTP destroys dopaminergic cells of SNPC A9. This is an irreversible and progressive illness. There may be faster tremors (4-6HZ) and reflexes may be increased.

Reversible Drug Induced Parkinsonism

Reversible drug induced Parkinsonism may be caused by the following drugs:
- Phenothiazines
- Haloperidol
- Metoclopramide
- Reserpine
- Bradykinesia
- Acute extrapyramidal effects
- Cervical dystonia.
- No tremors.

Toxic Causes

Manganese
- Manganese miners
- Welders.

Clinical Features

- Severe depression is an early feature
- Loss of postural reflexes
- Frequent falls.

Post Hypoxic

This is often associated with myoclonus, and choreoathetosis.

Methanol

- Akinetic rigid presentation
- MRI shows increased T2 signal of the striatum.

Mercury

- Akinetic rigid presentation
- Choreoathetosis
- Peripheral neuropathy.

Tremor

It is an involuntary movement which is rhythmic in nature due to synchronous contractions of agonist and antagonist muscles.

Differential Diagnosis

- Physiologic
- Pathologic: Parkinson's disease
  - Tremor of peripheral nerve origin
  - Drugs
  - Cerebellar disease
  - Midbrain (rubral)
  - Wilson's disease
  - Toxins
  - Metabolic.

Pathologic Tremor

- Resting tremor
- Attenuated with intention characteristics of basal ganglia diseases.

Benign Essential Tremor

Clinical Features

- Family history is positive in 20% cases.
- There is an increased incidence of Parkinson's disease.
- Affects men and women equally.
- Autosomal dominant mode of inheritance.
- Affect is on chromosome 3Q13 HS1 - BP 3 genes.
- Rare at rest.
- Kinetic.
- May be associated with poor fine movement.
- Responds to alcohol, gabapentin, benzodiazepines, beta-adrenergic blockade.

Clinical Variants

Primary writing tremor:
- Affects writing in isolation.
- Possibly initiated by hand position.
- Family history is positive in 30% cases.

Voice tremor:
May be associated with spasmodic dysphonia combined with resting and postural tremor.

Wilson's Disease

General Features

- Autosomal recessive chromosome 13 Q/4
- Presents with liver signs, and psychiatric manifestations.
- There may be presence of Kayser-Fleischer ring, which affect the cornea.

Associated Neurologic Signs

- Dystonia
- Chorea
- Myoclonus
- Dysarthria
- Cerebellar signs
- Seizures.

Pathology

- Atrophy of putamen
- Glial modification
- Diffuse atrophy of cerebellum and cerebral cortex.

Dystonic Tremor

- Jerking tremor like movements
- Pain in distribution of the affected segment.

Action Tremor

- Cerebellar disease
- Best seen on finger nose finger testing.

Clinical Features

- Specific cerebellar lesions produce tremors of specific type.
- Lateral cerebellar hemispheric lesion: Extremity tremor, tremor of the head and trunk, Lesion of the vermis or fastigial nucleus.
- Rubral tremor: Lesion near the red nucleus.

Usual pathologies of cerebellar tremor are sequale of severe head trauma, coma or interruption of the Dento - Thalmo - rubral pathway by vascular lesions. The stroke usually involves top of the basilar artery, branch of the posterior cerebral artery.

Drugs Causing Tremor

- Alcohol withdrawal
- Amphetamines
- Antihistamines
- Valproate
- Anticholinergics
- Calcium channel blockers.
- Beta-adrenergic agonists.
- These tremors are usually postural and bilateral.
- The tremor seen after alcohol withdrawal is increased by activity and emotional stress.

Metabolic Causes of Tremor

- Carbon monoxide
- Parkinje cell loss due to heat stroke
- Mercury poisoning

Psychogenic tremor is seen often, the hallmark being changing characteristics of the tremor, increases with attention, response to placebo and spontaneous remission. It often has abrupt onset and sporadic course.

Chorea

Chorea is characterized by the presence of sudden, irregular brief involuntary, irregular movements of the extremities, face or trunk.

Causes

- Hereditary
- Huntington's disease.

General Features

- Autosomal dominant mode of inheritance
- Genetics: Chromosome 4 (CAG Repeat (37-86) range for disease,
- Low frequency in Japan, Black population of USA.
- The age of onset, age of death, and rate of progression have inverse correlation with CAG repeat length.

Clinical Onset

- Juvenile (4-19 years)
- Late onset at greater than 50 years.

Pattern of clinical presentation:
- Common form: Chorea first presentation
- Hypotonia
- Dementia - frontal lobe features
- Chorea may precede or follow dementia
- Juvenile form: Gene is inherited from affected father.
- Bradykinesia
- Rigidity
- Seizures
- Movements persist during sleep.

Late onset:
- Uncommunicative
- Cognitive dysfunction
- Dystonia
- Dysphagia.

Diagnosis

Laboratory features:
CT shows enlarged lateral ventricles and flattening or absence of the caudate nucleus.

PET shows hypometabolism of the caudate nucleus and putamen.

Other Hereditary Causes of Chorea

- Wilson's disease
- Hallervorden - Spatz disease
- Abetalipoproteinemia
- Alzheimer's disease, late onset.

Infectious Causes of Chorea

- Sydenham's chorea
- Behçet's disease
- Subacute sclerosing pan encephalitis
- Encephalitis
- Systemic lupus erythematosus.

Drug Induced

- Levodopa
- Phenytoin
- Amphetamines.

Metabolic/Toxins

- Chorea gravidarum
- Birth control pills
- Renal failure
- Hypernatremia
- Hypo - Hypercalcemia.

Hemichorea

- Usually due to vascular lesion of the contralateral subthalamic nucleus, thalamus or caudate nucleus.
- Rarely complication of thalamotomy or tumor.

Sydenham's Chorea

- Following streptococcal infection with consequent rheumatic fever and heart valve - mitral/aortic involvement
- Familial tendency
- May resolve spontaneously within 3 to 6 months.
- May be associated with behavioral abnormalities and seizures
- Chorea gravidarum: Primarily distal extremities are involved and occur for first time during pregnancy. May be seen in women taking oral contraceptive pills.
- Associated with abnormal tongue movements.

Tardive Dyskinesia

Most common drugs include metoclopramide, prothiazine, and dopamine receptor antagonists.

Abnormal movements occur during drug treatment and after drug withdrawal.

Clinical Features

- Abnormalities of gait, trunk, posture, rhythmical involuntary movements of the tongue, face and jaw.
- Choreioform movements of the extremities.
- Athetosis.

Akathisia

Akathisia is associated with complex stereotyped movements of the extremities and trunk.

Clinical Features

- Subjective sensation of restlessness with inability to stay still.

- Movements present throughout the day.
- Causes include drugs, Parkinson's disease, obsessive compulsive disease, Tourette's syndrome, etc.

Athetosis

Definition

Slow writhing, involuntary, large amplitude movements that primarily involve distal extremities. It is often associated with facial grimacing and dysarthria.

Writers Cramp

- Form of dystonia
- Family history is positive in a large percentage of patients. They may have relatives with dystonia.
- Usually occurs in second to fourth decade.
- This may present with painful cramps while writing.
- To start with symptoms may be seen after prolonged writing.
- It is a form of focal dystonia.

Other Forms of Focal Dystonias

Other forms of focal dystonia include the following:

Idiopathic Torsion Dystonia

Genetics:

- Autosomal dominant inheritance involving the chromosome 9 1TDI gene.
- Incidence 1/15000 persons.
- Usually begins as focal action dystonia; about 70% cases may be generalized.

- Some family members have focal dystonia and others have generalized dystonia.
- Starts in distal legs in form of difficulty in walking due to dystonic movements of the foot, which affects plantar flexion and inversion.

Spasmodic Torticollis

- Affects sternocleidomastoid and trapezius muscles resulting in tonic or clonic contractures of neck muscles.
- Some sensory tricks such a touching the forehead may block specific dystonias.
- Associated with postural tremors and essential tremors.
- Usually progresses for 5 years and then stabilizes.

Blepharospasm

Bilateral spasmodic blinking may interfere with vision, sensory tricks such as singing, talking, reading, etc. Chewing may increase or decrease its occurrence.

Myoclonus

Definition: Very rapid brief shock like jerks precipitated by sensory stimulation. May originate anywhere in the neuraxis cortex, cerebellum, basal ganglia, and brainstem.

Physiologic Myoclonus

- Occurs in normal individuals
- May be associated with hyperexcitable neurons of the cortex.

Sleep Myoclonus

Sudden movements occurring during sleep or sleep transition.

Nocturnal Myoclonus

- Repetitive stereotyped dorsiflexion of the toes and foot.
- Associated with restless leg syndrome
- Occurs during Non REM sleep
- Increased incidence in patients with daytime drowsiness and insomnia.

Other forms of physiologic myoclonus include those induced by:

- Anxiety
- Exercise
- Hiccough.

Epileptic Myoclonus

- Epileptic myoclonus is a type of myoclonus occurring in a patient with seizure disorder.
- It is probably of cortical origin.
- May be an independent manifestation of seizure disorder or accompany other manifestation such as tonic clonic features.
- Cardinal features are: Photosensitive epileptic myoclonus; and myoclonic absences.
- These are seen in older children.

Childhood Myoclonus

- Infantile myoclonus
- Lennox-Gastaut syndrome
- Familial myoclonic epilepsy

Specific Diseases

Lundborg-Baltic myoclonus:

- Onset: 7 to 10 years age
- AR inheritance

Clinical features:
- Attempted movement
- Light noise, touch
- Seizures
- Dementia
- Spasticity
- Ataxia.

EEG: Generalized spike and wave discharges with photosensitivity.

Lafora Body Diseases

- Chromosome 6 Q gene

Clinical onset:
- Childhood or adolescent onset
- Seizures
- Dementia
- Myoclonus
- Death occurs 2 to 10 years after the onset of symptoms.

Tay-Sachs GM2 Gangliosidosis

- AR inheritance: Hexosaminiadase A enzyme deficiency
- Cherry rod spot in the retina
- Dementia
- Blindness
- Deafness
- Stimulating sensitive myoclonus.

Toxins that cause myoclonus:
- Bismuth
- Mercury

Palatal Myoclonus

Rhythmic contractions usually 60 to 180 / minute of the palate and pharyngeal innervated musculature, persists in sleep.

Asterixis

Asterixis is characterized by sudden brief loss of postural tone, usually while extension of the wrist and hand. It could be related to lesions of medial frontal cortex, internal capsule and rostral midbrain. Some of the medical conditions in which asterixis may be encountered include the following:
- Hepatic failure
- Renal failure
- Respiratory failure
- Hyperosmolar states.

Tic Disorders

Consists of:
- Eyeblinking
- Nose twitch
- Shoulder shrug
- Jerking extension of the head.

Differential Diagnosis

- Levodopa
- Carbamazepine
- Phenytoin
- Phenobarbitone.

Gilles de la Tourette's Syndrome

- Autosomal dominant
- 1 to 10 per ten thousand children prior to age 22.

- Coprolalia
- Copropraxia.

Associated disorders: Attention deficit hyperactivity disorder and obsessive compulsive disorders.

- *Pathology:* Atrophy of caudate and putamen.

Restless Leg Syndrome

- There may be positive family history in some patients.
- The patient may have irreversible urge to move the legs.
- May be associated with paresthesias, dysthesias, and motor restlessness.

Associated Medical Conditions

- Vitamin deficiency
- Pregnancy
- Uremia
- Mechanism: Dopaminergic mechanism is possible.

Autosomal Dominant Ataxia

Clinical Features

- Ophthalmoplegia
- Optic atrophy
- Peripheral neuropathy
- Pyramidal and extrapyramidal signs.
- Genetic heterogeneity
- Onset from 3rd to 5th decades.

ABNORMAL MOVEMENTS ASSOCIATED WITH CEREBELLAR DISORDERS

For various disorders affecting the cerebellum which can result in abnormal movements, refer to Chapter number 6.

8 The Cerebral Hemispheres

The brain is that part of the CNS which lies within the cranial cavity. It consists of six major parts.

1. Cerebrum
2. Diencephalon
3. Midbrain
4. Pons
5. Medulla oblongata
6. Cerebellum.

Cerebrum is the largest part of the brain. It consists of two large hemispheres: the left and right cerebral hemispheres, which occupy the anterior and middle cranial fossae and the supratentorial region of posterior cranial fossa. Each cerebral hemisphere consists of a surface layer of gray matter called cerebral cortex and a central core of white matter. In the basal part of the latter are located large masses of gray matter known as basal ganglia. The two hemispheres are separated from each other by a deep median longitudinal fissure called longitudinal cerebral fissure. The corpus callosum, which interconnects the corresponding cortical areas of the two cerebral hemispheres, lies in the floor of the fissure. The surface of cerebral cortex is convoluted. It has a series of elevations, the gyri, which are separated by shallow depressions, the sulci or deep grooves called fissures. Important sulci include the central sulcus, and lateral sulcus. Sulci vary in their appearance and position, but some are constant. The median and lateral sagittal sections of the brain are shown in Figures 8.1 and 8.2 respectively.

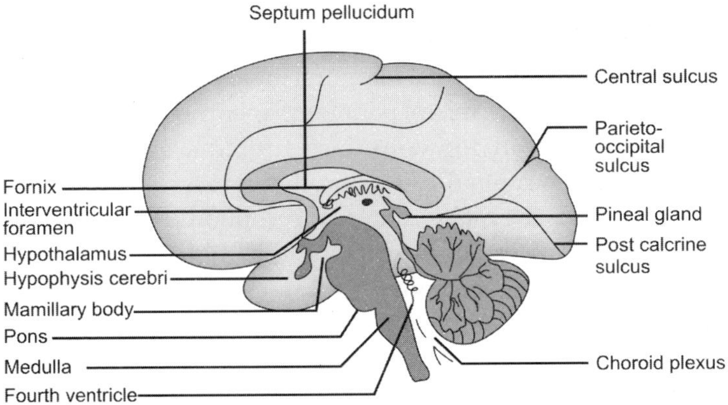

Fig. 8.1: Median sagittal section of the brain

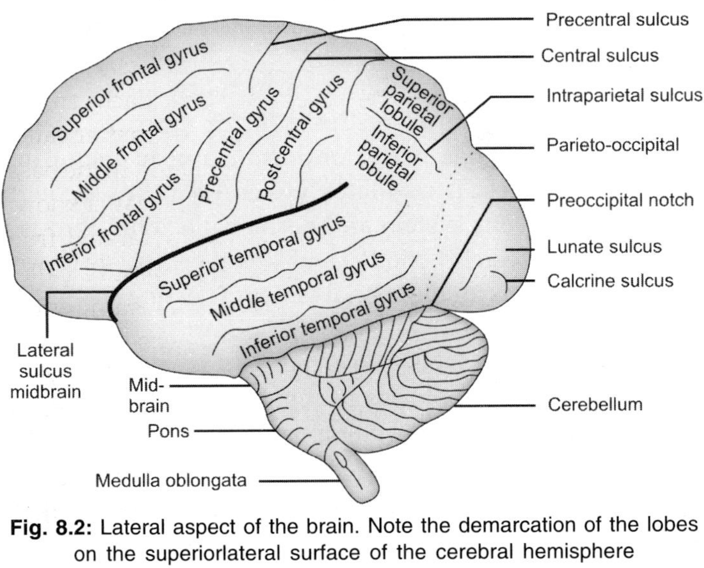

Fig. 8.2: Lateral aspect of the brain. Note the demarcation of the lobes on the superiorlateral surface of the cerebral hemisphere

The cerebral hemisphere is divided into 4 lobes. These include: Frontal lobe, anterior to central sulcus and above the lateral sulcus; parieteal lobe, which is posterior to the central sulcus and above the lateral sulcus; occipital lobe, which is behind a line extending from parieto-occipital sulcus to the preoccipital notch and the temporal lobe, which is below the lateral sulcus and in front of parieto-occipital notch. The frontal lobe is important for voluntary functions, motivation, aggression, emotional effects, and awareness of self. The parietal lobe is the major center for reception and evaluation of all sensory information except for smell, hearing and vision. The occipital lobe is responsible for reception and integration of visual input.

The temporal lobe receives and evaluates input for smell and hearing and plays an important role in memory. Limbic lobe lies between telencephalon and diencephalon. It is ring-shaped and is associated with basic survival instincts. It also provides ability to store and retrieve information and is particularly important for short-term memory.

The hypothalamus is the inferior portion of the diencephalon. It has many important nuclei including mamillary bodies. It regulates visceral activity through autonomic nervous system and hormonal activity through the hypophysis cerebri. Medial and lateral geniculate bodies form relay stations for the special senses of hearing and vision respectively.

Pineal gland is a small area of the diencephalon and along with habenular nuclei forms the epithalamus. Pineal gland has important role in controlling onset of puberty. It is also involved in sleep-wake cycle.

The habenular nuclei have olfactory and limbic connections. **Subthalamus** is a small area of diencephalon that lies between the thalamus and the midbrain. It contains several tracts and subthalamic nuclei which are associated with the basal ganglia and are involved in controlling motor functions.

Thalamus: The thalamus consists of the two thalamic nuclei, which form the largest mass of diencephalon and are separated by the cavity of third ventricle.

Thalamus forms an important relay station for all sensory impulses except smell, visual and auditory stimuli and appreciation of pain and touch. The thalamic neurons send projections to the sensory area of the cerebral cortex. The thalamus also integrates motor functions, retaining impulses from the cerebellum and corpus stratum to the motor area of the cerebral cortex. Its connections with limbic area influence mood, emotions and behavior.

VENTRICULAR SYSTEM AND CSF IN CNS

The ventricles of the brain are four in number – two lateral ventricles, a third ventricle and a fourth ventricle (Figs 8.3 and 8.4). The two lateral ventricles are separated from each other by the septum pellucidum extending from the corpus callosum and fornix. The third ventricle is a narrow slit- like cavity of the diencephalon. The two ventricles are connected with the third ventricle by the interventricular foramina called the foramina of monro. It communicates with the fourth ventricle via cerebral aqueduct of midbrain. The fourth ventricle is continuous with the central canal of the spinal cord. The central canal has a small dilatation at its inferior end, the terminal ventricle. The cerebrospinal fluid is formed by the choroid plexuses and passes through the roof of the fourth ventricle into the subarachnoid space around brain and spinal cord.

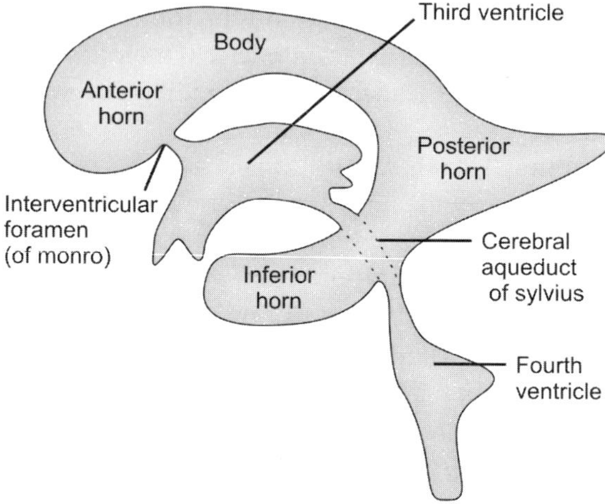

Fig. 8.3: Ventricular system lateral view

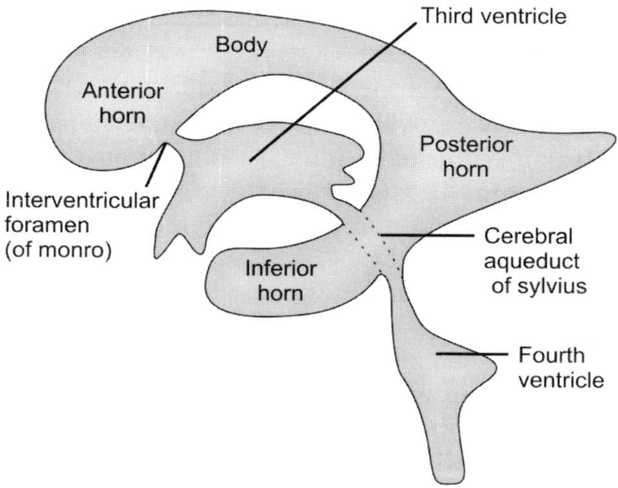

Fig. 8.4: The ventricles of the brain

The brain is surrounded by three protective membranes called meninges. From within outwards these are (1) Pia mater (2) Arachnoid mater (3) Dura mater. The subarachnoid space between the pia and arachnoid mater contains cerebrospinal fluid and the major arteries.

General

Clinical, anatomical correlation as well as functional studies with PET, SPECT, functional MRI, magnetoencephalography, and atomic force microscopy reveal that distributed networks form the anatomical basis of behavioral neurology.

A lesion in varied areas of the brain may destroy a functional network which may cause a specific deficit. Nevertheless, it is still useful to assign major functions to specific anatomical areas of the brain.

Many anatomical, pathological, and clinical correlates have withstood the test of time, but underlying mechanisms have changed. Therefore, discharge from one area of the brain, if severe and persistent, may damage its homologous area or another part of distributed network by Glutamate – NMDA excitatory mechanism, induction of apoptosis from intracellular calcium disregulation or neural plasticity induced by early response of genes.

FRONTAL LOBES

Left Frontal Lobe

Functions of the frontal lobe include the following:

1. Behavior
2. Abstract thinking
3. Planning
4. Executive function.

Aphasias

Expressive and conductive aphasias occur with damage to area 44. Lesions in the frontal operculum and area triangularis cause change in hand writing and many grammatical mistakes may also occur. Various apraxias occur with frontal lobe lesions. Apraxia is defined as inability to perform an individual or sequential task with normal motor, normal sensory and coordinative abilities. Some of these apraxias include eyelid opening apraxia, constructional apraxia, visual neglect, gait apraxia, and undue fatigue at the completion of the task.

Behavioral deficit which may be subtle includes the following:

1. Inability to copy facial movements.
2. Difficulty following multiple commands.
3. Inability to follow consecutive hand movements.

The Right Frontal Lobe

The functions of the right frontal lobe are involved with emotional and inhibitory control over limbic system. They are also associated with disinhibition of personal behavior, hygiene, sexual conduct, Confabulation, and inappropriate jocularity "witzelsucht".

Dorsolateral Prefrontal Cortex

It is important as a store of knowledge. Its functions range from solving problems of immediate environment, to performing behavioral functions requiring multiple sequences. It is important in memory retrieval.

The frontal eyefields are located in the prefrontal cortex which initiate saccadic eye movements and are important in occular fixation. It may present as pseudodepressed syndrome manifesting in the form of psychomotor inhibition, apathy, lack of drive and reduced emotional reaction.

Supplementary Motor Cortex

Damage to the supplementary motor cortex causes:
- Aphasia
- Disturbed coordination of movements on both sides while performing tasks such as walking, swinging phase, etc.
- Generation of movement may also be affected
- Mirror movements may be seen.

Orbitofrontal Cortex Damage

The damage causes psychopathic behavior, which is evidenced by:
- Disinhibition
- Lack of concern for the effects of behavior.
- Inappropriate sexual behavior.
- Retrograde amnesia (in bilateral lesions).
- Confabulations in medial orbital frontal lesions.
- Mania.

THE PARIETAL LOBE

The parietal lobe is central to somatosensory function, awareness of the body parts in space and gravitational awareness, that is awareness of the body within the vertical plane. Various areas in the parietal lobe serve specific functions. Lesions of area 3b, primary parietal cortex or post-central gyrus cause the sensation of heaviness in the extremities; lesions of area 3b1 diminish the person's ability to appreciate texture of the object, and that of area 2 affects the ability to perceive information regarding the "shape" and to receive information from deep tissues, joints, fascia and tendons.

General Sensory Functions of Parietal Lobe

These include the following:
- Two-point discrimination
- Graphesthesia
- Stereognosis
- Point localization.

Posterior Superior Parietal Cortex

This area is concerned with:
- Manipulation or active touch.
- Gesture representations.
- Inability to recognize objects (area 7).

Inferior Parietal Lobe

This area is concerned with:
Memory or recognition of spatial position.

Right Parietal Lobe

The lesions in this area result in the following:
- Visuospatial processing
- Denial of illness
- Left visual inattention
- Constructional apraxias
- Dressing apraxias
- Inability to discriminate between unfamiliar faces.

- Decreased short-term memory, and topographic disorientation.

Left Parietal Lobe Function

Gerstmann Syndrome

This syndrome is characterized by the presence of following features:

- Right left confusion
- Inability to cross the midline
- Finger agnosia
- Conduction aphasia
- Alexia without agraphia.

Conduction aphasia (area 39, 40, 41) is seen due to the disconnection between the Wernicke's and Broca's areas and damage to the arcuate fasciculus.

Parieto-occipital Junction – Balint's Syndrome

This is characterized by the presence of following features:

- Optic apraxia – undershooting of an object.
- Deficit in visual scanning.
- Color anomia
- Anomic aphasia
- Ideational apraxia.

The Temporal Lobe

Function

- Receptive speech, particularly Wernicke's area.
- The inferior temporal gyrus is essential for object recognition, while the middle temporal gyrus visual area is important for recognition and tracking of moving objects.

- Middle temporal gyrus area is important for registration and consolidation of short-term memory.
- Personality and its substrates is sub served by temporal lobe through its projections to the limbic system.

Left Temporal Lobe

Lesions of the left temporal lobe can produce the following conditions:

- Wernicke's aphasia
- Sensory conduction aphasia
- Short-term memory loss
- Color anomia
- Nominal aphasia

Right Temporal Lobe

Anterior temporal lobe lesions produce:

- Anxiety/panic attacks
- Delirium
- Amnesia
- Various deficits due to hippocampal damage like:
  - Hunger auras
  - Spatial information deficit.
  - Pathological crying.

Bitemporal Lobe Diseases

This includes the Klüver-Bucy syndrome, which is characterized by the presence of following:

- Hypersexuality
- Sham rage
- Severe memory deficits.

Differential diagnosis of KBS includes the following:
- Herpes simplex encephalitis
- Head trauma
- Radiation to pituitary tumors
- Temporal lobectomy

Amygdala

Clinical features due to the lesion of amygdala include the following:
- Freezing response
- Slow contralateral turning
- Automatism including smacking of the lips or chewing.
- Ictal fear associated with anxiety or feeling of impending doom.

Cingulate Gyrus

It comprises of mamillary bodies, the mamillothalamic tract, the hippocampus and anteroventral thalamic nucleus. It is involved in herpes simplex encephalitis, paraneoplastic encephalomyelitis and seizure disorders.

Clinical Features in Lesions of Cingulate Gyrus

Anterior Cingulate Gyrus
- Deficit in motivation
- Bradykinesia.

Posterior Cingulate Gyrus
- Learning and memory impairment
- Pain on one side of the body.

In general, the signs seen in cingulate gyrus lesions are disorders of obsessive compulsive behavior, and hemineglect of contralateral space.

Occipital Lobe

The occipital lobe is central to all aspects of vision. Stimulation of area 17 of calcrine cortex in the awake patients produces non-colored, non-moving flashes of light with geometric designs. Stimulation of area 18 and 19 produces geometric figures in the contralateral visual field, where as the stimulation of areas in junction of temporoparietal/occipital cortex causes visual distortion and complex visual hallucinations. Besides, various forms of dysphasias are encountered; color naming may be absent in lesions of fusiform gyrus, and there may be visual agnosia in bilateral lesions of the junction of temporal/occipital cortex.

Disorders of Complex Visual Processing

Visual Agnosia

This is the disorder of higher function wherein a normal nonaphasic patient with normal visual perception is unable to recognize visual stimuli.

Prosopagnosia

It is a form of visual agnosia, characterized by an inability to recognize previously known human faces and to learn new ones. Recognition through other sensory channels is intact.

Classically, this is manifested in form of vascular lesions involving posterior cerebral arteries, or space occupying lesions and has also been observed in epileptic patients.

Cortical Blindness

This occurs due to bilateral damage to both visual cortices and to the optic radiations. They are euphoric, unable to see, deny blindness, may have confabulate vision and normal pupillary response.

Alexia

Alexia without agraphia is also known as "word blindness". These individuals have normal visual acuity and can recognize nonverbal stimuli. They cannot read, but can copy what they cannot read. The lesion involved is extensive and disconnects both visual association cortices from the dominant language area. Usually corpus callosal lesion combined with a lesion of the left occipital cortex causes disconnection of visual associative cortex with language area.

Disorders of Color Perception

Color Naming

- Matching of colors is normal.
- Inability to name colors.
- No dysphasia.
- No defect of color perception.
- Right hemianopia.
- Pure alexia.
- Lesion may be in the left hemisphere between occipital and temporal lobe lesion for right homonymous heminopia plus it may also be in the geniculate body, optic radiation or visual cortex.

Disorders of Spatial Analysis

Visual Disorientation

Features

- Optic ataxia (inability to grasp an object using visual guidance)
- Ocular apraxia
- Inferior quadrantic visual field defect.

Cause

- Thrombosis in the water shed zone between anterior and posterior cerebral arteries and middle cerebral artery (Balint's syndrome).
- Brodmann's area 7, 19 and 39 may be involved.

Disorders of Arousal

The ascending reticular activating system and posterior thalamic nuclei interact to determine the state of arousal. Reticular activating system which starts in the medulla receives projections from spinothalamic tracts and all major special senses, dorsal pons, periaquectal gray and intralaminar nuclei of the thalamus are the subcortial components. The intralaminar nuclei project to the cerebral cortex.

Causes

Vascular disease:

- Thalamic hemorrhage
  - Basal ganglia infarction.
- Epidural/subdural hematoma
- Brain tumor
- Metabolic causes
  - Hepatic failure
  - Abscess.

THE BASILAR SYNDROME

- Bilateral thalamic infarction.
- *Cerebral herniation* that causes stupor due to cingulate gyrus herniating under falx.

- Unilateral temporal lobe swelling.
- Third nerve palsy is an early sign.
- Posterior fossa lesion.
- In children most often tumors.

Other Causes

- Sleep apnea
- Delirium (drugs, toxins metabolic, disorders)
- Locked in syndrome.
- Akinetic mutism.

Akinetic Mutism

Patient lies mute in a state of disordered arousal and he is neither able to initiate nor respond to verbal stimulus.

Lesion is usually in the base of frontal lobe and could be due to trauma, tumors, or aneurysm of anterior cerebral artery.

Chronic Vegetative State

General Features

- Unconsciousness
- Inability to respond to verbal or painful stimuli.

Causes

Lesions may be in reticular activating system, periaqueductal gray matter or cortex. The various causes are as follows:

- Trauma.
- Basiliar artery stroke.
- Raised intracranial pressure.

MEMORY

Amnesia: Anterograde amnesia is the inability to learn new material. Retrograde amnesia is inability to remember events prior to injury. Confabulation is the use of fabricated verbal responses concerning questions regarding recent events.

Korsakoff's Syndrome

Korsakoff's syndrome occurs due to thiamine deficiency (alcohol, pernicious vomiting, renal dialysis).

Clinical Features

- Ataxia
- Ophthalmoplegia
- Nystagmus
- Peripheral neuropathy
- As the acute confusional state clears, there may be residual deficit in acquiring new information Confabulation.
- Retrograde amnesia.
- Anatomically, the cause includes bilateral lesions of the mamillary bodies, and hypothalamic nuclei.

Dorsal Medial Nuclei of Thalamus

Hypothalamic tumors: Amnesic syndrome has been observed in cases of hypothalamic tumors particularly, those surrounding the floor and walls of third ventricle.

Thalamic lesions:
- These lesions may be produced due to thalamatomy, thalamic infarcts, etc.
- These lesions are often associated with anterograde and retrograde amnesia.

- Bilateral fornix lesions and cingulate lesions cause amnesia and confabulation similar to Korsakoff's psychosis.
- Surgical resection of temporal lobe may also inhibit new learning, and inability to recognize faces.

Transient Global Amnesia

This is characterized by anterograde amnesia, which lasts for about 3-24 hours. Retrograde amnesia may accompany first few hours of the syndrome of global amnesia. There are no accompanying neurological deficits. Recovery usually occurs rapidly.

Causes

Causes include the following:
- Posterior cerebral artery thrombosis
- Migraine
- Headache
- Seizures.

Causes of amnesia may include the following:
- Head trauma, epilepsy, electroconvulsive therapy
- Drugs – benodiazepines
- Huntington's disease
- Depression.

Confusional State

General features:
- There is a failure of attention
- No localizing signs other than tremor, asterixis, and myoclonus

- Thought and skilled movements are affected.
- The stream of thought is affected by frequent intrusions of competing thoughts and sensations.

Clinical Features

- Distractibility.
- Lack of vigilance.
- Inability to maintain coherent stream of thought.
- Patients are disoriented, and may have memory deficits.
- Dysgraphia, constructional apraxia and poor judgment.
- Lack of insight, apathy.

Causes

- Toxic metabolic encephalopathy.
- Multifocal brain lesion.
- Head trauma.
- Epilepsy.
- Space occupying brain lesion.
- Multifocal brain disease.
- Alzheimer's disease
- Meningitis
- Encephalitis
- Anoxia
- Subdural hematoma.

Focal Brain Lesion

Lacunar Infarction

This usually occurs due to infarctions in the parietal and inferior prefrontal regions of the right hemisphere.

Aphasia and Apraxia

Broca's Aphasia

- Difficulty in initiating and articulating speech.
- Comprehension is abnormal.
- Writing is abnormal.

Wernicke's Aphasia

Patient cannot comprehend or repeat spoken language. Reading and writing are affected. Accompanying features include lack of insight, apraxia and superior quadrantic defect.

Conduction Aphasia

- In these cases, the comprehension is preserved.
- Repetition is impaired.
- Naming is impaired.
- Writing demonstrates omissions, spelling errors, and altered sequences of words and letters.
- Conduction aphasias are produced due to lesion in the supramarginal gyrus and arcuate fasciculus.

Transcortical Motor Aphasia

- Difficulty in initiating speech.
- Difficulty in naming.
- Well preserved comprehension.
- Writing is poor.

Transcortical Sensory Aphasia

Similar to Wernicke's aphasia, there is poor comprehension but in contradistinction to Wernicke's aphasias the patient has preserved repetition. They cannot read or write. Concomitant signs include hemisensory deficit visual field defects, and hemiparesis. This lesion is most commonly produced due to the damage to angular gyrus or second and third temporal gyrus.

Global Aphasia

Global aphasia is produced as a result of the damage to frontal and parietotemporal language area due to carotid or middle cerebral artery occlusion. The person cannot initiate speech, follow commands, read, write or repeat names. There may be concomitant right hemiplegia.

Dysarthria

General Features

- There is an articulation defect.
- The individuals can express themselves in written language.
- They can fully comprehend written and spoken language.
- Speech is grammatically intact.
- Lesions of the medial frontal cortex or supplementary motor area or cingulate gyrus may simulate this defect.

Pure Word Deafness

The patient is unable to interpret spoken language, but can identify non-verbal sounds. They can read, and write. However, they can neither comprehend spoken language nor repeat it. The anatomic lesions are in Heschl's gyrus. The second localization is bilateral damage to the mid-portion of the superior temporal gyrus. Cortical deafness occurs with bilateral damage to Heschl's gyrus and their connections. Patients are aware of words and sounds but cannot interpret them.

Alexia without Agraphia

Clinical Features

- Inability to comprehend written language.
- Words spelled out loud are recognized.
- Letters written on palm are recognized.
- Words constructed with blocks when palpated with hands are recognized.
- Patients may have impairment or loss of color vision.
- The patients are unable to name colors although they can recognize them.
- Thrombosis of left posterior cerebral artery resulting in infarction of the left occipital lobe and the splenium of the corpus callosum may give rise to agraphia.
- Thrombosis of dominant middle cerebral artery or its distal branches may also give rise to loss of ability to read and write due to the infarction of parietal lobe.
- There may be accompanying mild hemiparesis, hemisensory loss, and anomic aphasia.

Paralexia

Paralexia is associated with substitution of words or syllables when reading out aloud.

Agraphia

- Aphasia associated with abnormal writing
- *Anterior frontal syndrome*: Large poorly constructed words, misspelling and omission of functions, words and endings.

Types of Agraphia

Visual–spatial agraphia

- Patient is able to formulate correct letters and words but has great difficulty in arranging them correctly on page and having them progress from one line to the next.
- Seen in dominant hemisphere lesions or may form part of Gerstmann's syndrome.
- All aphasics have difficulty in finding specific words in spontaneous speech and also in naming.
- This is found in dementia, raised intracranial pressure, acute confusional states and psychoses.
- Two forms of specific defects are mentioned: Word selection anomia wherein patient is unable to name an object on confrontation by any sensory modality but can describe its use and can select when it is named by the examiner lesion is Brodmann's area 37 (Temporo-occipital junction of the dominant hemisphere).

Semantic Anomia

This is characterized by inablility to both name the object or to select it when it is named.

A. *Syndrome of calculating impairment*
   Aphasic Acalculia
   - Not able to utilize numbers as a language entity
   - Unable to write numbers or comprehend numbers correctly.
   - Usually seen in all aphasics and follows damage to the dominant hemisphere.

B. *Visual Spatial Acalculia*
   - Understands numbers and computational signs.

- Inability to place numbers in correct space.
- Lesions are in non-dominant hemisphere at parieto-occipital junctions.

APRAXIAS

It is defined as inability to perform an individual or sequential function with intact motor, sensory or coordinative abilities.

Lesions in different areas of brain may result in different forms of apraxias:

Ideational Apraxia

The patient is unable to correctly carry out the correct sequence of a common task although each separate task can be correctly performed. For instance, when given a cigarette, the patient may be unable to show how he would smoke the cigarette. The whole act of removing the cigarette from the packet, inserting into the mouth and lighting it may be affected. Lesion is in parietal area 5 and 7.

Constructional Apraxia

This is characterized by the inability to construct the copy of a visually presented object with blocks or by drawing. Both right and left parietal lobe lesions cause the defect although right parietal lobe lesions are more commonly affected than left sided lesions. Associated feature with left parietal lobe lesions may include fluent aphasia.

Dressing Apraxia

The patient is unable to dress himself when given the garment. It is commonly produced due to bilateral occipitoparietal lesions. It may also be seen in demented or confused patients.

Callosal Apraxia

Corpus callosum lesion: There may be inability to perform a simple command with left hand although right hand is able to perform.

Gait Apraxia

- There is inability to initiate swing component of gait.
- Feet may not have firm grasp of the floor.
- This apraxia is seen in normal pressure hydrocephalus, and in conditions wherein locomotor center, cerebellar peduncles – pontine nuclei input and output may be affected by lesions such as tumors, vascular disease or cysts.
- Often basal ganglia disease and lacunar strokes present with difficulty at the time of diagnosis and should be considered in differential diagnosis of true gait apraxia resulting from disorders mentioned.

9 Cranial Nerves

CRANIAL NERVE-I

OLFACTORY NERVE

Important Features

The fibers of this nerve are classified as special somatic afferent fibers. They carry sense of smell from olfactory epithelium of the nose which is derived from ectoderm. The olfactory nerve penetrates the cribriform plate of the ethmoid bone to synapse on the olfactory bulb (Fig. 9.1).

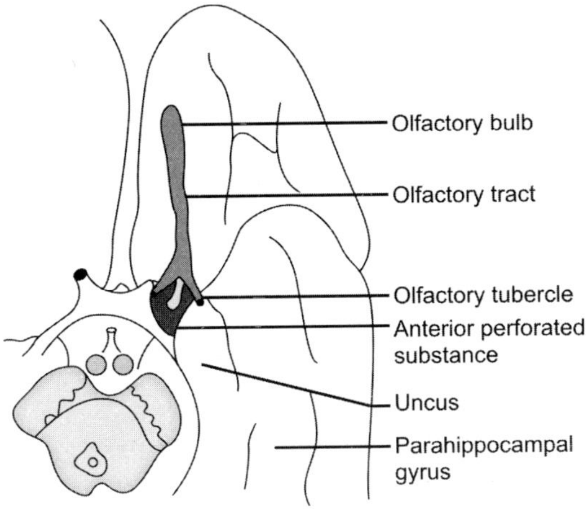

Fig. 9.1: Olfactory structures (anterior part of the brain)

The axons form the olfactory tract. The olfactory tract divides into lateral and median olfactory stria. The lateral striae project to ipsilateral piriform lobe of temporal cortex (primary olfactory cortex) with projections to amygdala, septal nuclei and hypothalamus.

Unilateral loss of smell is caused by lesion of the olfactory bulb, tract or striae.

Anosmia

Anosmia is commonly caused by trauma and fractures of cribiform plate of the ethmoid bone. Some of the other causes of anosmia are described below:

1. Closed head injury without fracture (olfactory filaments tear)
   - Basilar skull fracture (discrimination in sense of smell, detection is preserved).
   - Korsakoff's syndrome.
   - Thalamic lesion.
   - Alzheimer's disease.
   - Parkinson's disease.
   - Other neurodegenerative diseases.
2. Tumors
   - Olfactory groove meningiomas.
   - Glioma of the frontal lobe.
   - Carcinomatosis of the meninges.

Olfactory Hallucinations

Olfactory hallucinations are primarily caused by:

- Primary cortical (olfactory) injury
- Direct interruption of the olfactory pathway
- Complex partial seizures.

CRANIAL NERVE-II

OPTIC NERVE

Rods and cones originate from the retinal epithelium. Rods and cones then project to bipolar cells, which project to ganglion cells; further projection is to lateral geniculate body or superior colliculus. The visual pathway is described in the Figure 9.2.

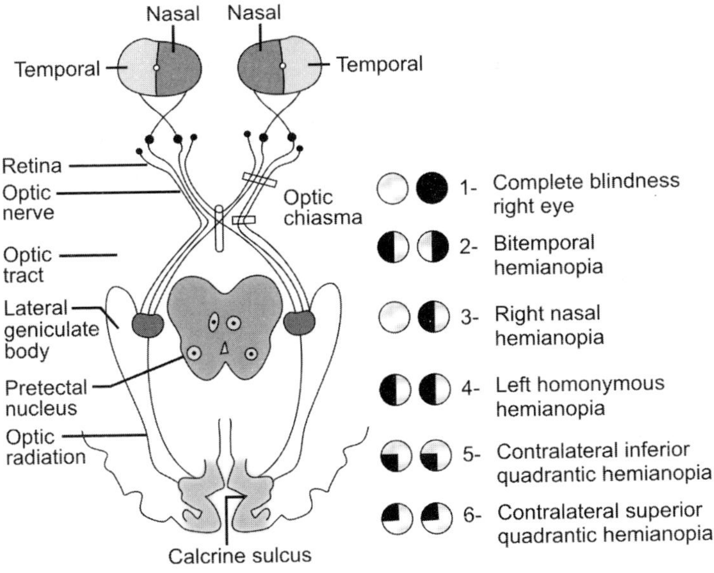

Fig. 9.2: Visual pathway and visual field defects 1–6

Optic Nerve and Optic Chiasm

Blood supply: There occurs an area of watershed between central retinal artery (Ophthalmic) and posterior ciliary arteries (external carotid). In 80% of individuals, this area is above the dorsum sellae. In 5% of cases, it is prefixed, overlying the anterior margin of sella and in the remaining percentage of population, it lies over the diaphragm sella.

The Optic Radiations

The optic radiations are composed of fibers from the lateral geniculate body entering the occipital cortex. They comprise of an upper bundle and a central bundle.

Vascular Supply of the Visual Pathways

Vascular supply of the optic nerve: Near the optic chiasma, the optic nerve is supplied by the carotid and anterior cerebral artery. Proximally, it is supplied by the ophthalmic artery.

Optic tract: The optic tract is supplied by posterior communicating artery, posterior cerebral artery and anterior choroidal artery.

Lateral geniculate body is supplied medially by anterior choroidal artery and laterally by posterior choroidal artery.

Optic radiations are supplied by middle cerebral artery and posterior cerebral artery.

Vascular Disease of the Optic Nerve

This is usually due to central retinal artery emboli from carotid atheroma, arch of the aorta and heart valves.

They are birefringent, yellow cholesterol plaques (Hollenhorst plaques) which lodge at branch points of secondary and tertiary arteries

Ischemia of the chiasm occurs either due to pressure of the aneurysm or clipping.

Another important condition affecting the optic nerve is delayed effect (1-5 years) of X-RT which affects the endothelium.

Hereditary Disease of the Optic Nerve

- Retinitis pigmentosa
- Glaucoma
- Hereditary sensory motor neuropathy
- Familial spastic paraplegias
- Leber's hereditary optic atrophy.

Immune Mediated Optic Atrophy

Causes of immune mediated optic atrophy include the following:

- Multiple sclerosis
- Devics disease
- Associated with chronic inflammatory demyelinating peripheral neuropathy
- Associated with adult subacute sclerosing panencephalitis
- Postimmunization.

Tumor

- Lymphoma: Mass effect-optic nerve head affected by compression.
- Melanoma: Malignant
- Rebinoblastoma-childhood illness.

Orbital Complications of Sinus Disease

- Frontal sinusitis due to mucocele, empyema, etc.
- Maxillary sinusitis characterized by bone or optic nerve involvement.

- Ethmoidal sinusitis due to mucocele, or suppuration
- Sphenoidal sinusitis: Optic neuritis, cavernous sinus thrombosis.

Optic Nerve Disease due to Vitamin Deficiency and Toxins

- Vitamin B_{12} deficiency
- Thiamine deficiency
- Multiple vitamin deficiency

In elderly patients, supplementation with thiamine is of therapeutic value.

Optic Nerve Disease due to Drugs and Toxins

- Drugs (e.g. ethambutol, isoniazid, etc.)
- Tobacco
- Alcohol amblyopia.

Ischemic Optic Neuropathy

Infarction of the disk is characterized by the presence of following features:

- Sudden loss of vision
- No recovery
- Flame shaped hemorrhages in the edematous region of the disk
- Papilledema.

Clinical Signs

- Fat veins
- Dilatation of capillaries at the surface
- Loss of venous pulsation.
- Slit hemorrages of the disk capillaries.

- Loss of disk margin
- Optic atrophy
- Sharp disk margins
- Loss of lamina cribrosa
- Decreased visual acuity
- Decreased cup disk margin ratio.

Empty Sella Syndrome

- Extension of the subarachnoid space through the diaphragm sella
- Normal volume of the sella

Empty sella syndrome is often associated with pseudotumor cerebri or arachnoid cysts.

Clinical Features of Importance

- Headache
- Blurring of vision
- Diplopia
- Obese women
- Occasionally CSF rhinorrhea.

CRANIAL NERVES III, IV, VI (OCULOMOTOR, TROCHLEAR, ABDUCENS)

Oculomotor Nerve

Nucleus (Midbrain): The two nerves then emerge from the midbrain between the cerebral peduncles. They then splay on as they pass anteriorly, lying between the posterior cerebral arteries and superior cerebellar arteries, while running parallel to the posterior communicating arteries until they enter the cavernous sinus lying between two layers of dura that forms lateral wall of the sinus. It enters the orbit through the superior orbital fissure and divides into two main branches: The upper branch supplies the eyelid and superior rectus muscle, whereas the lower branch supplies the medial rectus, the inferior rectus and inferior oblique and via the ciliary ganglion, it also supplies the pupil.

Blood supply: Small arteries from the posterior cerebral and basilar arteries. The orbital portions arise from recurrent branch of the ophthalmic artery.

Causes of 3rd Nerve Damage

Trauma

- Head trauma between posterior cerebral and the superior cerebellar arteries.
- At the tentorial edge
- In the cavernous sinus.

Neoplasms

- Midbrain tumors: Glioma, medulloblastoma, metastatic lesions, etc.
- Pituatory adenoma may affect the nerve as it spreads into cavernous sinus.
- Nasopharyngeal tumors - Affect the nerve in cavernous sinus.
- Instrinsic tumors of the IIIrd nerve.
- Schwannoma.
- Neurofibroma.

Muscle Disease Affecting Third Nerve

- Oculopharyngeal dystrophy
- Myotonic dystrophy

- Mitochondrial disease: Kearns - Sayre syndrome - complete ophthalmoplegia, heart block, hearing loss, and diabetes.

Neuromuscular Disease

Acquired myasthenia
- Pupil spared
- Asymmetrical ptosis.

Botulinium toxin
- Bilateral ptosis
- Bilateral dilated pupils

Eaton-Lambert syndrome is a neuromuscular disease associated with impaired muscle strength on exercise, and asymmetrical ptosis.

Infections

Third nerve palsy may occur with herpes zoster, measles, HIV, syphilitic basal meningitis, tuberculous meningitis, mucormycosis, *Cryptococcus* infection, etc.

Systemic Disease

Diabetes mellitus: Pupils are usually spared; painful or painless ophthalmoplegia.

Wernicke's-Korsakoff's syndrome: This usually occurs in association with thiamine deficiency: Encephalopathy and neuropathy are associated features.

Other Causes

- Immune mediated
- Miller fisher variant: Guillain-Barré syndrome.

- Ophthalmoparesis.
- Areflexia, ataxia are concomitant features.
- Chronic inflammatory demyelinating polyneuropathy.

IVTH NERVE: TROCHLEAR NERVE

Supranuclear control is entirely crossed nucleus at the level of inferior colliculus in the brainstem and fibers crossover at the level of periaqueductal gray matter and the superior medullary velum so that right nerve originates in the left trochlear nucleus. It has a long intracranial course as it enters the cavernous sinus. It enters the orbit through superior orbital fissure and crosses the third nerve. It supplies the superior oblique muscle.

Lesions of Trochlear Nerve

Lesions of trochlear nerve can occur due to the following causes:

- Vascular lesions can occur as part of superior cerebellar artery stroke.
- Trauma severe head injuries - brainstem distortion, orbital fracture may damage IVth nerve.
- Arteritis: Diabetes, granulomas.
- Post-traumatic, intracavernous aneurysm.
- Systemic disease, cavernous sinus infection, carcinomatosis.
- Neuromuscular junction disease.
- Congenital and acquired myasthenia gravis.
- Lambert-Eaton syndrome.
- Infections like syphilis, herpes zoster, mucormycosis, etc.

VITH NERVE: ABDUCENS NERVE

Nucleus: Ventral pons

It enters the cavernous sinus next to carotid artery and may be involved within inferior petrosal sinus as it courses through Dorello's canal.

Lesions of Abducens Nerve

Lesions of the abducens nerve can occur due to the following causes:

Head trauma:
- Fracture at the base of the brain.
- Fracture of the temporal bone.
- Fracture of the orbital wall.

Neoplasms:
- Glioma
- Meningioma
- Acoustic neuroma
- Carcinoma of meninges
- Lymphoma
- Breast, thyroid, lung metastasis.

Infective Lesion

Gradenigo's syndrome: Facial numbness; masseter, pterygoid and temporalis weakness; contralateral loss of pain and temperature below the clavicle; contralateral hemiparesis. Pathogenesis: This syndrome usually occurs due to secondary thrombosis of short circumferential artery, branch of the basilar artery.

Other Infections

- Tuberculosis
- Mucormycosis
- Cryptococcosis.

Immune Mediated

- Miller-Fisher variant of GBS
- Multiple sclerosis
- Chronic inflammatory demyelinating polyneuropathy.

CRANIAL NERVE-V: TRIGEMINAL NERVE

Trigeminal nerve arises from the middle of the pons. Its ganglion lies over the tip of the petrous bone in Meckel's cave where the nerve divides into three divisions: the ophthalmic, Maxillary and Mandibular divisions (Fig. 9.3).

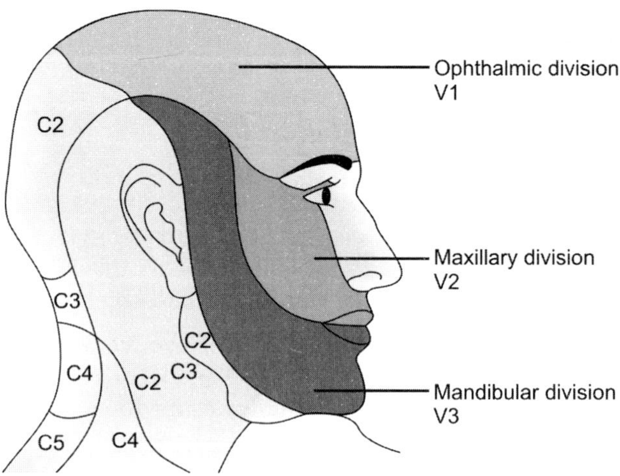

Fig. 9.3: Area of face supplied by trigeminal nerve

The Ophthalmic Nerve

The ophthalmic nerve lies below the sixth nerve in the lateral wall of the cavernous sinus. As it enters the superior orbital fissure it divides into three branches: the lacrimal nerve, frontal nerve and nasociliary nerve. The lacrimal nerve runs along the lateral rectus muscle to the lacrimal gland and supplies the skin over lateral eyelid and brow. The frontal nerve has two branches supratrochlear and supraorbital nerves which supply the skin of the forehead and scalp uptil the vertex. The nasociliary nerve has important autonomic and cutaneous functions and supplies the mucosa of the nasal cavity and tip of the nose, alae and vestibule. Its branches in the orbit carry pupillodilator sympathetic fibers and convey sensations from the cornea.

The Maxillary Nerve

The ganglion of the maxillary nerve lies in the lateral wall of the cavernous sinus and exits the skull through the foramen rotundum. It supplies the skin of the cheek, lateral part of the alae, lower eyelid and the mucous membranes of the cheek and the upper lip. It gives off the following branches: Meningeal branches, branches to sphenopalatine ganglion and the zygomatic nerve. Zygomatic nerve supplies sensation to the cheek alveolar nerve supply teeth, gums, palate, nasal wall, nasal septum, the lower eyelid and the skin of the upper lip. The pterygopalatine ganglion lies in the pterygopalatine fossa. It receives preganglionic parasympathetic fibers from the nervous intermedius (seventh nerve) and sympathetic fibers from the middle meningeal artery. Both groups of fibers are relayed to the lacrimal gland.

The Mandibular Nerve

It includes motor component of the nerve. The sensory branch- the meningeal branch accompanying middle meningeal artery supplies anterior, middle and lateral cranial fossae. Nerve to the medial pterygoid supplies the medial pterygoid, tensor tympani and tensor Veli palatani. The main nerve is joined outside the skull by motor root. It divides into anterior and posterior trunk. Anterior trunk supplies masseter, temporalis and lateral pterygoid. Buccal nerve supplies skin over the buccinators, mucous membranes of the cheek and posterior part of the buccal surface of the gum.

The posterior trunk gives rise to the following branches:

- Auriculotemporal nerve, which joins the facial nerve and supplies the skin over the tragus, helix, auditory meatus, tympanic membrane, and also gives secretomotor fibers to parotid gland.
- Lingual nerve: Tongue, the floor of the mouth and lower gums.
- Dental nerve - Lower lip, jaw incisors and canine teeth.

The motor component supplies mylohyoid and the anterior belly of the digastric muscle.

Testing for Corneal Reflex

Wisp of cotton with fine tip should be prepared. Patient looks up and to the side, with the examiner holding the patient's lower lid. The area between iris and cornea is stroked gently. Both eyes shut simultaneously if the corneal reflex is present.

Lesions of Trigeminal Nerve

Trauma

- Surgical trauma

- Head and facial trauma
- Dental treatment.

Tumors

- Trigeminal neuroma - Schwann cell origin.
- Numbness and paresthesia in the distribution of the nerve.
- Meningioma : Affects mandibular division
- Nasopharyngeal cancer.
- Lymphoma.

Vascular Syndromes

- Wallenbergs's syndrome - Posterior inferior cerebellar artery and vertebral artery occlusion.
- Cavernous sinus aneurysm
- Internal carotid artery aneurysm.

Systemic Disease

- Hypothyroidism
- Sarcoidosis
- Polyarteritis nodosa.

Trigeminal Neuralgia

Trigeminal neuralgia is associated with severe lancinating pain. Pain is most often unilateral and affects the mandibular division. There is usually refractory period between the attacks.

Triggering events include light touch of the affected division, chewing, swallowing, cold, etc.

Trigeminal neuralgia is usually idiopathic in nature, but occasionally in young patients, it may be manifestation of multiple sclerosis or vascular loop compression of the main trigeminal nerve at entry zone. The loop comprises of superior cerebellar artery, anterior inferior cerebellar artery and basilar artery.

Infections

- Gumma of the pons: Maxillary division is affected, mainly resulting in sensory loss. There may be paresthesia and numbness over the midface.
- Herpes simplex, herpes zoster
- Gradenigo's syndrome
- Purulent middle ear infection occasionally associated with lateral sinus thrombosis.
- Leprosy
- Other lesions - mainly structural
- Brainstem glioma
- Brainstem arachnoid cyst
- Syringobulbia.

Migraine Variants

Lower face V2 and V3 division paroxysal hemifacial pain responds to indomethacin. Cluster migraine, orbital, retro-orbital pain, Raeder's syndrome: VI distribution pain, photophobia, nausea, ptosis, miosis.

VIITH NERVE: FACIAL NERVE

Nucleus Pons

The nerve is primarily motor to the muscles of facial expression. It also conveys taste to anterior two-thirds of the tongue in the chorda tympani and taste from the palate through the nerve of the pterygoid canal. Vagus carries a cutaneous nerve from the seventh to the external ear. The cell bodies of the sensory root lie in the geniculate ganglion. The greater petrosal nerve arises from the geniculate ganglion, carrying taste fibers from the palate. Lesser petrosal nerve conveys secretomotor fibers in the auriculotemporal nerve to the parotid gland. Nerve to the stapedius: This nerve supplies the stapedius muscle. Posterior auricular nerve supplies the muscles of the ear and occipital belly of occipitofrontalis. Submandibular ganglion preganglionic fibers are derived from the superior salivatory nucleus in the brainstem. The innervations to the muscles of facial expression can be separated into the muscles of the upper part of the face and muscles of the lower part of the face. The supranuclear input responsible for the movement of the upper facial musculature is a bilateral input from the cortex to the nucleus. The supranuclear input responsible for the movement of the lower facial musculature is only a contralateral input from the cortex to the facial nucleus. If the patient with facial droop can move the upper facial muscles (wrinkle the forehead) the lesion is supranuclear on the contralateral side. The lesion probably is somewhere in the contralateral corticobulbar tracts above the facial nerve nucleus.

If the patient cannot voluntarily move any muscle involved in facial expression either of upper or lower facial musculature the lesion is localized to the facial nucleus or the peripheral facial nerve on the ipsilateral side.

Bell's Palsy

Bell's palsy is one of the most common neurological disorders. It is acute lower motor neuron facial palsy. There may be aching pain around the ear. Predisposing factors for Bell 's palsy include diseases like diabetes, hypertension, etc. In approximately 80% of cases, the recovery occurs within 2-6 weeks; steroids are helpful if started in adequate dose of 30 mg and continued for two weeks after the onset.

Herpes Zoster Syndrome

Also known as Ramsay Hunt syndrome, this syndrome is caused by herpes zoster virus.

Clinical Features

- Eruption of vesicles around external auditory meatus and over the mastoid process.
- Lower motor neuron facial palsy.

Upper Motor Neuron - Facial Weakness

Causes

- Internal capsule infarction
- Lacunar infarction
- The pathogenesis is due to atheroma.
- Tumors in the cerebral hemisphere such as glioma, meningioma can also give rise to upper motor neuron facial palsy.

Head trauma and infections such as tuberculosis, basal meningitis, syphilis, affects the facial nerve at the nucleus fascicle or in its peripheral distribution. The associated feature is affectation of 5th and 6th nerve palsies. In cavernous sinus thrombosis, 5th, 6th and 7th nerves are affected together.

CRANIAL NERVE-VIII: COCHLEAR AND VESTIBULAR NERVE

This nerve has two components:

- *Auditory:* Afferents from the cochlea.
- *Vestibular:* Afferents from the saccular and utricular macula.

Core system for audition:

This comprises of:

- Central nucleus of the inferior colliculus
- Components of the medial geniculate
- Primary auditory cortex.

Vestibular System

Afferents:

- Superior nucleus (semicircular canals)
- Lateral nucleus (SCC)
- Medial nucleus (SCC)
- Vestibular efferents
- Medial longitudanal fasciculus.
- Medial vestibular tract
- Lateral vestibulospinal tract
- Cerebellum receives afferents from inferior and medial nuclei
- Fastigial nucleus
- Reticular formation receives afferents from lateral reticular nucleus.

Clinical Features

General:

- Decreased perception of tone or speech: lesion central to the oval window.

- Sensorineural loss
- Greater difficulty with high pitched sound
- Loss of speech discrimination
- Tinnitus.

Causes of Tinnitus

- Tumors: Glomus jugulare tumor
- Arteriovenous malformation
- Labyrinthitis
- Brainstem lesions.

Lesions causing sensorineural deafness:

- Cerebral lesions (Area 41, 42, 43)
- Bilateral lesions of the auditory cortex
- Temporal lobe epilepsy
- Peripheral nerve lesions.

Cochlea

Clinical features due to cochlear lesions

- Deafness
- High frequency hearing loss
- Tinnitus.

Causes

- Basal skull fracture
- Syphilis
- Cerebellopontine angle tumors.

Acoustic neuroma: It originates from the vestibular portion of VIIIth nerve in the internal auditory canal. It is characterized by progressive, sensorineural hearing loss; vertigo; ipsilateral unsteadiness; weakness of V, VI, and VII nerves; weakness, and loss of taste of anterior 2/3rd tongue and sometimes decreased corneal reflex. If the tumor extends posterioly, cranial nerve IX may be involved resulting in dysphagia, and absent pharyngeal reflex. Involvement of cranial nerve X may result in hoarseness, where as the involvement of XI cranial nerve may result in the weakness of muscles like trapezius, and sternomastoid. Romberg's sign and finger nose finger test may be positive. Nystagmus, with horizontal, rotatory fast component of nystagmus to the opposite side may be present.

Differential diagnosis of peripheral vestibular disturbance:
- Acute severe vertigo
- Absent calorics on the affected side
- Acute labyrinthitis.
- Meniere's disease
- Episodic severe vertigo
- Fluctuating sensory neural hearing loss. Bilateral in 50% patients.
- Systemic causes of severe vertigo
- Congenial syphilis
- Viral, bacterial labyrinthitis, diabetes mellitus, hypothyroidism
- Cardiac arrhythmias
- Ramsay Hunt syndrome - Herpes zoster
- Anemia
- Hypoglycemia
- Vascular causes of severe vertigo
- Vertebrobasilar insufficiency
- Lateral medullary syndrome
- IXth and Xth nerve involvement vertigo, dizziness, nausea, vomiting.

Bickerstaff's Migraine

Features
- Short duration loss of consciousness
- Dizziness
- Dysarthria, ataxia
- Tingling of the hands
- Cerebellar infarction, hemorrhage.

Hereditary Hearing Loss

Syndromatic causes:
- Mitochondrial encephalopathy (MELAS)
- Pigmentary retinal dystrophy
- Deafness
- MERFF syndrome (Mitochondrial encephalomyopathy with ragged fibers)
- Kearns Sayre syndrome.

IXTH AND XTH CRANIAL NERVES: GLOSSOPHARYNGEAL AND VAGUS NERVES

Glossopharyngeal Nerve

Nucleus

Brainstem: Nerve emerges dorsal to the inferior olivary nucleus in close relation to the cranial nerves X and XI.

The only muscle supplied by this nerve is stylopharyngeus. This cannot be tested clinically.

Sensory fibers: Afferents from posterior 1/3rd of tongue, tonsils, and nasopharynx.

Taste fibers from the posterior 1/3rd tongue, traveling via the petrous ganglion, ultimately terminate in the nucleus tractus solitarius.

Clinical Features of IXth and Xth Nerve Lesions

- Taste sensation is affected
- Decreased gag reflex
- Decreased salivary secretion from the parotid gland.

Causes of Lesions to the IXth and Xth Nerve

Glossopharyngeal neuralgia (IXth nerve):
- Idiopathic
- Secondary to structural lesions
- Stabbing unilateral pain
- Hacking cough
- The attack of severe pain is usually triggered by swallowing, talking, coughing, etc.
- Associated features include bradycardia, syncope, etc.

Other lesions of IXth nerve:
IX nerve may also be involved in the following lesions:
- Tumors such as glomus jugulare
- Metabolic disease
- Peripheral nerve or neuromuscular junction lesion
- Diphtheria
- Acute and chronic inflammatory demyelinating polyneuropathy
- Tabes dorsalis
- Retropharyngeal lesions
- Abscesses
- Aneurysms
- Adenopathy.

Vagus Nerve

The Nuclei

Dorsal nucleus - contains motor and sensory fibers.

The nucleus ambigus: gives origin to fibers controlling the striated muscle of the pharynx and the intrinsic muscles of the larynx.

The nucleus of the tractus solitarius is shared with glossopharyngeal nerve and receives fibers from the taste buds of the epiglottis. The spinal nucleus of the 5th nerve receives afferent fibers from the pharynx and larynx.

Since the motor distribution of the vagus comprises the nerve supply to the palate and the vocal cords, weakness of the palate causes nasal regurgitation of food and nasal speech. The paralyzed side of the palate is pulled to the intact side when the patient says "Aah". Also paralysis of the vocal cord leads to hoarseness, loss of volume of the voice and inability to cough.

Causes of Lesions of Xth Nerve

Bilateral upper motor neuron lesion as a result of damage to the cortical representation in the precentral gyrus gives rise to clinical features of pseudobulbar palsy which manifests as emotional incontinence, pathologic laughter and crying, spastic dysarthria, gag reflex.

Medullary lesion can occur due to motor neuron disease, primary and metastatic tumor, Wallenberg's syndrome, posterior fossa tumor, idiopathic meningitis, glomus jugulare tumor and meningioma.

CRANIAL NERVE-XI

Accessory nerve arises from the upper cervical and lower medullary anterior horn cells and supplies sternocleido-mastoid and trapezius muscles. It exits the cranial vault via jugulare foramina. If left spinal accessory nerve is cut, the resulting weakness of the sternocleidomastoid causes inability of the patient to turn the head to the right. The left trapezius also becomes weak and the patient is unable to shrug the left shoulder.

CRANIAL NERVE-XII: HYPOGLOSSAL NERVE

The hypoglossal nerve is the motor nerve to the tongue. The tongue muscles in addition to moving the tongue from side to side also move it up and down and in and out. Unilateral damage to the nerve supply leads to wasting, weakness and fasciculation of that side of the tongue. The most important cause of injury to the XII nerve is the neurofibroma of the twelfth nerve. The right hypoglossal nerve innervates the right tongue muscles; it thus acting alone pushes the tongue to the left. Similarly the left hypoglossal nerve innervates left tongue muscles; it thus acting alone pushes the tongue to the right. Together these muscles act to push the tongue forward. If there is a lesion in the left hypoglossal nucleus, the right hypoglossal muscles acts unopposed. Therefore the tongue deviates to the left; in other words the tongue deviates towards the affected side.

Jugular foramen syndrome: Since, the cranial nerves, IX, X, and XI exit the cranial vault through the jugulare foramen, damage to the nerves due to tumor, basal meningitis, etc. compromises the function of these nerves. Symptoms include loss of taste sensation in the posterior two thirds of the tongue, paralysis of the vocal cords, palate and pharynx and paralysis of the trapezius and sternocleidomastoids.

10 The Autonomic Nervous System

The autonomic nervous system (ANS) controls the activities of the heart, blood vessels, glands and smooth muscle throughout the body. It can be divided on the basis of the anatomical situation of the connector cells and fibers. Thus, the connector cells in the brain, their axons in the cranial nerves specified and their related ganglionic neurons constitute the cranial division of the system. The connector cells in the thoracolumbar region, their axons in the corresponding ventral roots, their subsequent ramifications and their ganglionic neurons constitute the sympathetic nervous system (Fig. 10.1). The sacral connector cells, their axons in the sacral ventral roots and all their related ganglionic neurons constitute sacral autonomic division (Fig. 10.2). The cranial and sacral divisions in physiologic terms have complimentary actions. If stimulated, they produce antagonistic actions. Under natural conditions, the two systems act synergistically. The main neurotransmitter in the autonomic nervous system is acetylcholine (ACh), which acts as the neurotransmitter for all preganglionic neurons and for the parasympathetic postganglionic neurons.

It has two types of receptors: Nicotinic and muscarinic. Nicotinic receptors mediate fast responses and are found mainly in the ganglia. Muscarinic receptors mediate slower responses and are found mostly throughout the autonomic

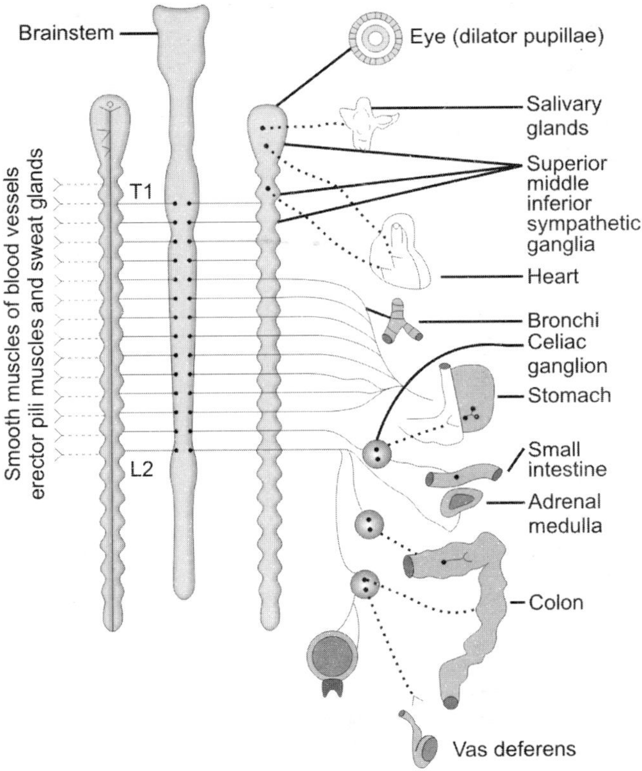

Fig. 10.1: Sympathetic nervous system. Postganglionic sympathetic fibers are shown by interrupted lines

effector tissues. Five subtypes (M1 - M5) of muscarinic receptors have been identified and cloned.

Norepinephrine is the neurotransmitter for most sympathetic postganglionic fibers. Adrenergic receptors are divided into alpha (Alpha 1, and Alpha 2) and beta (Beta 1, Beta 2 and Beta 3) types and are localized in a variety of

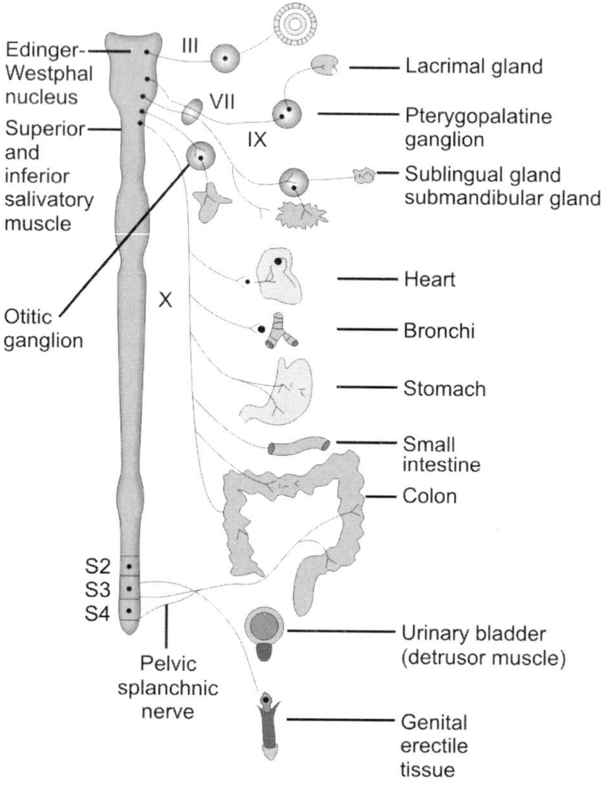

Fig. 10: 2: Parasympathetic nervous system (craniosacral outflow)

autonomic effector tissues. Various other neurotransmitters have been identified, which are neuropeptides and may act as neuromodulators in autonomic signaling. Examples include substance P, somatostatin, vasoactive intestinal peptide, enkephalins, and oxytocin.

NUCLEUS SOLITARIUS

Nucleus solitarius is an important nucleus situated in dorsomedial medulla receiving input from forebrain nuclei, brainstem and diencephalon. The afferents controlling cardiac rhythm, motility, peripheral vascular tone, respirations, and secretion, terminate in this nucleus. Efferents from nucleus solitarius end on the neurons of reticular formation which in turn project to the ventral horn of the spinal cord. It also sends efferents to the vagus and hypothalamic and limbic system. It thus plays a vital role in maintenance of body homeostasis. Recent studies in rats indicate that nucleus solitarius plays a critical role in transmission of signals from the peripheral nervous system to the hypothalamus that process memory for emotionally significant experiences, mostly involving pain and temperature.

DISEASES ASSOCIATED WITH AUTONOMIC NERVOUS SYSTEM

- Peripheral neuropathies – diabetes
- Vitamin B_{12} deficiency, alcoholism, paraneoplastic syndromes.
- Inherited peripheral neuropathies
- Riley-Day syndrome
- Fabry's disease
- Porphyria
- Amyloidosis
- Some spinocerebellar degeneration.

Systemic Disease

- Systemic lupus erythematosus

- Rheumatoid arthritis
- Guillain-Barré syndrome
- **Lambert-Eaton myasthenia syndrome: LEMS is an antibody mediated autoimmune disease**. It is a paraneoplastic syndrome characterized by dry mouth, impotence, constipation, blurred vision, impaired sweating, difficulty in micturition, and variation in heart rate and blood pressure.
- **Subarachnoid hemorrhage, cerebral infarction and cardiac arrhythmias** are often associated with features of autonomic dysfunction due to an imbalance between sympathetic and parasympathetic influences on the heart. In brain injury, dysautonomic manifestations are frequent, resulting in marked agitation, hyperthermia, tachycardia, and hypertension. This syndrome is often designated as diencephalic seizures or **paroxysmal autonomic instability with dystonia**.
- **Parkinson's disease**: Autonomic dysfunction in Parkinson's disease is common, resulting in symptoms like salivation, sweating, bladder and bowel dysfunction, and orthostatic dizziness. These autonomic dysfunctions are thought to be due to a central cause.

GENETIC CAUSES OF DYSAUTONOMIA

Riley-Day Syndrome

General Features

- Hereditary autosomal recessive disorder.
- It affects people of **Ashkenazi Jewish** extraction.
- It affects the development and survival of sensory, sympathetic and parasympathetic neurons.

- Frequency is 1 in 3600 live births of Ashkenazi Jews
- **Gene identified as 1 KBKAP gene on the distal long arm of Chromosome 9.**

Clinical Signs

- *Absent papillae of tongue*
- *Depressed patellar reflexes*
- Absent skin response to scratch and histamine injection.
- Relative insensitivity to pain and temperature.
- Sural nerve biopsy: Diminished myelinated and non-myelinated axons.

Fabry's Disease

General Features

- X-linked recessive metabolic disease.
- Deficiency of the lysosomal enzyme **alphagalactosidase.**
- Result of the enzyme deficiency is the storage of glycolipid, ceramide trihexoside in the body cells including skin, kidneys, cardiovascular and pulmonary systems, and blood vessels.
- Many patients develop myocardial infarction before 50 years of age.
- Posterior cerebral circulation strokes are common.
- **Mutation in the alpha galactosidase** gene has been identified.

Other Clinical Features

- Diminished sweating.
- Reduced cutaneous skin response.
- Reduced tear and saliva production.
- Abnormal cardiovascular response.

REM AND NON REM SLEEP

Autonomic Changes

During REM sleep sympathetic activity of the splanchnic and renal circulation is decreased and activity of skeletal muscle is increased. In NREM sleep – slow phases of sleep – there is hypotension and bradycardia, which become pronounced as this sleep phase progresses from stage I to stage IV. However, REM sleep is associated with large transient increases in blood pressure. Thus, slow wave sleep during the early phase of sleep cycle provides a protective effect on the cardiovascular and cerebrovascular systems. During REM sleep such protective effects disappear. This phenomenon may explain why cardiovascular and cerebrovascular events occur more frequently in the early mornings after awakening.

11 Cerebrovascular Diseases

The cerebral hemispheres are supplied by the terminal branches of the carotid and basilar arteries (Fig. 11.1). There are efficient collaterals between different branches.

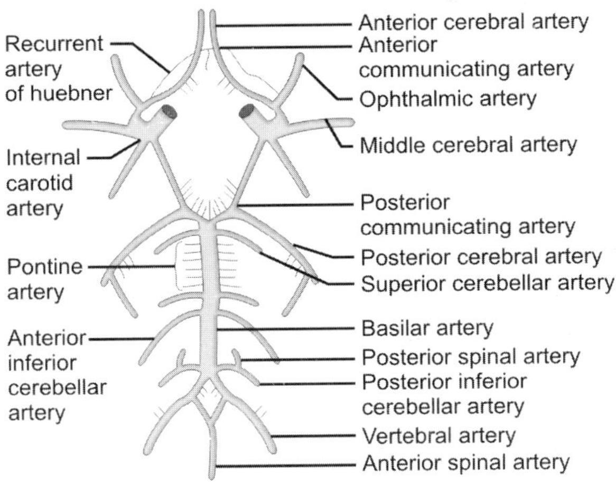

Fig. 11.1: Blood supply to the cerebral hemispheres

THE ANTERIOR CEREBRAL ARTERY

Anatomy: The anterior cerebral artery arises from the internal carotid artery in the cavernous sinus. It divides into two vessels: the pericallosal and callosomarginal arteries which supply the parasagittal cortex including motor and sensory cortex controlling leg. There is an inconstant branch of the anterior cerebral artery called recurrent artery of Huebner which contributes to the descending motor fibers in the internal capsule and supply cranial nerve nuclei and the arm on the opposite side.

The two anterior cerebral arteries are joined by anterior communicating artery which is a collateral to the opposite hemisphere.

THE MIDDLE CEREBRAL ARTERY

The MCA originates at the bifurcation of the internal carotid artery, just above the cavernous sinus. In the sylvian fissure it trifurcates. It is here, that there is narrowing of the lumen of the artery. There are about six to twelve branches of the MCA which penetrate deep into anterior perforated substance supplying basal ganglia and part of the internal capsule. These are the lenticulostriate arteries. The main divisions of the middle cerebral artery are precentral, central, posterior parietal and posterior temporal arteries. They supply the lateral surface of the hemisphere.

THE POSTERIOR CEREBRAL ARTERY

Posterior cerebral artery is formed by the bifurcation of the basilar artery in the interpendicular space. It gives branches which supply hippocampus and inferior medial surface of temporal lobe. It also gives rise to a series of penetrating vessels, which supply the dorsolateral brainstem, thalamus, sublenticular and retroventricular visual radiations. These are thalamogeniculate and thalamoperforating arteries. The main vessel continues as calcrine artery and supplies occipital cortex (visual cortex), with the exception of macular cortex at the tip of occipital pole which receives blood supply from the middle cerebral artery.

RISK FACTORS FOR ISCHEMIC STROKE

Primary

Ethnicity: Among people belonging to African, American and Asian ancestry, there is a tendency for increased accumulation of atherosclerotic lesions. Family history is often positive.

Secondary

Hypertension: Hypertension is commonly associated with accelerated atherosclerosis of large extracranial vessels, particularly arch of the aorta, carotid bifurcation, and large intracranial vessels. There may be accompanying stenosis and atherosclerosis of mouth of penetrating branches of the small vessels.

Concomitant risk factor is diabetes, specifically for infarction of thalamogeniculate and thalamoperforate arteries, and posterior inferior cerebellar arteries. It is also associated with lacunar state.

Smoking: It is a clear risk factor for involvement of extracranial and intracranial arteries.

RISK FACTORS FOR EMBOLIC STROKE

- Cardiac emboli.
- Artery to artery (intravascular) emboli.
- Cardiac arrhythmias (atrial fibrillation, tachyarrhythmias, bradyarrhythmias, etc.)

- Cardiomyopathy
- Mitral valve prolapse
- Valve replacement
- Infection
- Calcific aortic valve from bicuspid congenital defects
- Patent foramen ovale
- Thickening of valve cusps
- Myxematous degeneration of the chorda tendinea.
- Akinetic (postmyocardial) infarct
- Left ventricular aneurysms.

Hypertension

At any age there is positive linear relationship between both systolic and diastolic pressure and incidence of stroke. Even with a minimal reduction of blood pressure by 5-6 mm Hg, there is greater than 40% reduction in the incidence of all strokes, and 45% reduction in incidence of fatal strokes. Isolated systolic hypertension should be treated, especially if systolic blood pressure> 170 mm Hg. The risk of stroke can be significantly reduced by reducing systolic blood pressure by at least 10 mm Hg in the elderly.

Diabetes

Risk of stroke is increased to 2.5 to 3.5 times in diabetic patients in comparison to the controls.

Smoking

Smoking accelerates atherosclerosis, besides having an effect on platelet inhibitory factor. Cessation of smoking reduces the risk rapidly.

Hyperlipidemia

Elevated levels of total cholesterol and low density lipoproteins are independent risk factors for stroke development.

Effect of Cholesterol Reduction with Statin Drugs

Risk of stroke in those taking statin drugs was reduced by 30%. There was also reduction in mortality from stroke by 20%.

Oral Contraceptives

Use of high estrogen formulations in the past demonstrated an increased risk of stroke in women > 35 years of age.

Hyperhomocysteinemia

This is a risk factor for premature atherosclerotic peripheral vascular disease, myocardial infarction and stroke.

Silent Cerebral Infarction Associated with Coronary Artery Disease

By definition, silent cerebral infarction is an infarct demonstrated by CT or MRI without a history of stroke. 80% of those with coronary artery disease have silent cerebral infarcts. These infarcts are small, deep and present in the basal ganglia. They are usually less than 1 cm in size and occipital lobes may be disproportionately involved.

Alcohol

High alcohol consumption is associated with increased risk of stroke and intracranial hemorrhage.

Infections

Syphilis

Recently, accelerated atherosclerosis has been found to be associated in patients with cardiac transplantation (cytomegalovirus infection), as well as *Chlamydia pneumoniae*. Infections like HIV also confer significant risk for ischemic vascular disease.

Atrial Fibrillation

Patients with AF are at a four times higher risk of stroke.

Myocardial Infarction

With anterior wall MI the risk of stroke is 6%. With inferior MI, risk is about 10%. Most embolic events occur in the first two weeks after infarction.

Mitral Valve Prolapse

It is common among young women.

Complications are common in old age and in men. Associated features which predispose to stroke in MVP patients are mitral regurgitation and tricuspid valve prolapse.

Risk of Stroke Associated with Cardiac Surgery

In general, patients undergoing coronary artery bypass, valvular surgery or both have a risk of stroke between 2-6%.

TRANSIENT ISCHEMIC ATTACKS (TIA)

Embolic TIAs

Source

The source of emboli may be from an artery to artery or in form of clots and other material from the heart. They may occur as single episodes or as multiple episodes of amaurosis fugax. Predisposing factors for embolization include tight stenosis, lowered CBF (cerebral blood flow) and low systemic pressure.

Clinical Features

Clinical features may vary, but some features such as aphasia (pure receptive) are pathognomic of TIA. This is a characteristic feature resulting from the obstruction of temporoparietal branch of the inferior division of MCA due to atrial fibrillation.

Sometimes sudden headache or dizziness may be the only features. Also, isolated quadrantic hemianopia may be the only sign resulting from the obstruction of calcrine branch of PCA due to atrial fibrillation. Sometimes, subacute bacterial endocarditis may be heralded by TIAS to MCA territory.

Differential Diagnosis

Migraine: In this case, positive visual symptoms of scintillating or fortification scotomata show gradual evolution over 20 minutes and headache occurs after these symptoms. These features help in differentiating migraine from TIAS.

In case of TIAS, there are no auras, no loss of consciousness, no mental clouding and no TODD's paresis. Demyelinating disease with sudden onset, particularly which is associated with optic nerve involvement, may present with diagnostic difficulties. In these cases imaging is helpful in establishing the diagnosis.

Bickerstaff migraine: This may present with bilateral visual loss, paresthesia of the hands, perioral numbness, bilateral visual disturbance, dysarthria and loss of consciousness. These symptoms may be confused with brainstem stroke.

Age, sex and hereditary pattern help in differentiating migraine from Stroke (How?): This type of migraine was described in young women and the attacks occur usually prior to menstruation. In 60% of cases there is family history of migraine and the important clue is absence of motor weakness neuroimaging does not show changes of infarction in the brainstem. Headache invariably follows the Aura. Nevertheless in 50% of Brainstem strokes headache may be associated symptom and invariably ischemic changes are seen on MRI and PET scan in pons, midbrain and medulla. Angiographic study of posterior circulation TIAS particularly if they are of brief duration of less than ten minutes show in significant percentage atherosclerotic occlusive disease of the vertebral and basilar system.

Hypoglycemia, hepatic insufficiency: These may often present with clinical picture mimicking classical transient ischemic attacks.

Seizures: Seizures may be another differential diagnosis to be considered when tonic/clonic seizures occur as presenting feature, especially if the TIAS are in cerebral peduncle or internal capsule.

Diagnosis

Imaging studies

Imaging studies are helpful in diagnosis of TIA. T2 weighted images on MRI may demonstrate ischemic pneumbra.

MAJOR VESSEL STROKE

Carotid Occlusion

This causes weakness or paralysis of the contralateral arm face and leg. Head and eyes are deviated to the side of the lesion. Cerebral edema with Cheynes-Stokes respiration may supervene.

In cases where there is complete carotid occlusion, there may be no symptoms at all. This is especially so, if the process is gradual and if there is sufficient collateralization. Transient ischemic attacks may be presenting manifestation of preocclusive carotid disease. These may be ischemic orbital pain, optic atrophy, and bilateral or unilateral carotid bruits.

Acute Carotid Occlusion

Clinical features:

- Lethargy
- Fluctuating level of consciousness
- Seizures
- Horner's syndrome
- Periodic respiration
- Aphasia: Broca's > Wernicke's
- Contralateral Babinski's sign

Internal Carotid Artery Occlusion

Occlusion at the carotid siphon clinical features are:

1. Few episodes of amaurosis fugax
2. Leg > arm weakness
3. Slow progression of symptoms.

The Anterior Choroidal Artery Syndrome

It supplies caudal 2/3 of the posterior limb of the internal capsule, the posterior optic tract, cerebral peduncle, the uncus, portions of the thalamus and branch to choroid plexus.

Clinical Presentation

- Hemiparesis, hemisensory loss, hemianopia.
- Pure motor hemiplegia.
- Painful thalamic type syndrome (pain in the arm and leg; feeling of arm swelling)
- Hemiataxia
- Temporary sensory loss.

Higher function deficits
- Visual neglect
- Constructional apraxia
- Short-term memory loss
- Perseveration.

Pathogenesis of AChA occlusion
- Cardiac embolism
- Thrombosis – due to intracranial atherosclerosis
- Hyperviscosity states.

Anterior Cerebral Artery Infarction

Symptoms

- Paresis of Leg (foot) > arm
- Face, and tongue are spared
- Homolateral ataxia with cranial paresis
- Pure motor hemiparesis

- Psychomotor dysfunction: Anterior cerebral artery supplies the regions of the limbic system and basal ganglia, both of which are essential for integration of emotional aspects of movement and frontal lobe function. Loss of consciousness may be transient in ACA infarction.
- Akinetic mutisum – No emotional expression, inablity to initiate speech and movement.
- *Aphasia:* This may manifest in form of muteness, transcortical motor aphasia, transcortical sensory aphasia, and whispered speech.

Other signs and symptoms

- Urinary and fecal incontinence.
- Presence of grasp reflex.
- Ideomotor apraxia
- Impaired ability to imitate the examiner's movements with the left hand if infarction is in anterior corpus callosum.
- Left hand agraphia.
- Alien hand syndrome: In this syndrome, there is de-synchronization of movements of both hands. Unilateral damage to medial frontal lobe can trigger reaching and grasping movements in the contralateral hand. These movements are purposeful although patient may not perceive that he is in control of these movements. A patient may put a cigarrete in the mouth with the intact controlled hand (right hand) following which alien (left hand) may purposefully grasp the cigarrete and toss it away before it could be lit by the controlled hand. The lesion is in the mesial frontal lobe and corpus callosum.
- Pure motor hemiparesis

Middle Cerebral Artery Occlusion

Americans and Afro-Asians have higher incidence of MCA occlusion in comparison to the Europeans. Pathogenesis of middle cerebral artery occlusion is more often thrombotic than embolic.

Features

- Dominant hemisphere involvement
- Head and eye-deviation to the side of the lesion
- Lethargy
- Aphasia
- Superficial territory infarction
- Hemiparesis: faciobrachial > leg
- Contralateral pyramidal deficit
- Wernicke's aphasia
- Broca's aphasia
- Alexia without agraphia, conduction aphasia.
- *Deep territory middle cerebral artery territory infarction*: This causes internal capsule and basal ganglia infarction. Leg is more often involved, and there is absence of eye-deviation. These points help in differentiating deep territory infarction from superficial territory infarction.

Posterior Circulation Infarction

This can involve the following vessels:

- Arch of the aorta
- Innominate and subclavian arteries
- Vertebral, basilar, posterior cerebral vessels and their branches.

30% of emboli to the posterior circulation arise from the arch.

Subclavian Artery Stenosis

Subclavian steal syndrome: This results in inequality of pulses in the two arms. Blood pressure in the arm is lowered on the side of the stenosis. Other symptoms include claudication of the arm and brainstem symptoms.

Vertebrobasilar Infarction

This usually occurs proximal to the origin of the Vertebral Artery (VA) from subclavian artery. It is usually accessible to stenting and angioplasty and is commoner among the Caucasians in comparison to the Asians and African-Americans.

Clinical Features

- Dizziness
- Diplopia
- Dysphagia
- Hemiparesis
- Bilateral leg weakness
- Sensory loss on the trunk

Posterior Inferior Cerebellar Artery Infarction

This vessel supplies lateral medulla and the cerebellum.

Clinical Signs

- Lateral medullary infarction.
- Approximately 40% cases occur suddenly, whereas nearly 60% cases have a gradual onset.
- Cranial nerve abnormalities

- Dysphagia
- Hoarseness
- Nausea and vomiting
- Ipsilateral Horner's syndrome
- Hiccoughs
- Ipsilateral VII nerve dysfunction
- Blurred vision
- Diplopia
- Horizontal and rotatory nystagmus on the ipsilateral side
- Ipsilateral hemiparesis
- More often than not there is ataxia without weakness
- Ipsilateral limb ataxia.

Other Symptoms

- Headache, more often occipital/unilateral
- Autonomic dysfunction
- Cardiac arrhythmia
- Postural hypotension
- Sleep apnea.

Pontine Infarction

- In 1/3 of patients TIAS precede the stroke onset
- Pseudobulbar features, spontaneous laughing and crying.
- Tonic limb spasms.
- Lacunar infarctions: Dysarthria, vertigo, and gait abnormality.

MRI: The following features may be observed on MRI examination:

- Hypertensive vascular changes

- MRI shows increased T2 pontine signal
- Perivascular demyelination.

Specific clinical signs referred to Pontine infarction:
- Lateral pons: Horner's syndrome
- Ipsilateral taste loss
- Hemiataxia.
- Oculopharyngeal palatal myoclonus.

Basilar Artery Infarction

- Lacunar infarct
- Nonlacunar infarcts: Maximal diameter > 1.5 cm
- TIAS
- Diplopia, vertigo, blurred vision, ataxia, gait disturbances
- Pupillary abnormalities
- Hyperreflexia
- Bilateral Babinski's sign

Infarction due to Thrombosis

The following clinical signs and symptoms may be observed:
- Hemiparesis
- Dizziness
- Alternating level of consciousness
- Dysarthria
- Pseudobulbar features
- Emotional liability
- Paralysis of tongue
- Ocular bobbing, ocular dipping.
- VI and VII cranial nerve palsies with contralateral hemiplegia and paresthesiae.

Midbrain Infarction

Cardinal signs of midbrain infarction are isolated 3rd nerve palsy and pupillary abnormalities in nuclear lesions.

Weber's Syndrome

- Third nerve palsy and contralateral hemiplegia (Weber's syndrome).
- Supranuclear gaze palsy.
- Sensory symptom and signs and visual dysfunction if concomitant thalamic and occipital lobe signs are present.

Claude's Syndrome

Third nerve palsy and contralateral cerebellar dysfunction.

Benedict's Syndrome

It is characterized by 3rd nerve palsy plus abnormal movement.

It occurs due to the damage to the red nucleus, causing an interruption of the dentorubrothalamic tract from the opposite cerebellar hemisphere. The closer the infarction to the red nucleus, greater would be the tremor and postural fixation difficulty in the extremity.

Gaze palsies form important clinical manifestations of midbrain infarction.

Superior Cerebellar Artery Infarction

Superior cerebellar artery infarction results in destruction of:

- Periaqeductal gray matter
- Posterior commissure.

Median or Paramedian Infarction of the Upper Midbrain

Median or paramedian infarction of the upper midbrain results in the following:

- Conjugate vertical gaze palsy
- Upgaze paralysis
- Median longitudinal fasciculus
- Down gaze palsy
- Bilateral upper midbrain infarction associated clinical signs with gaze palsies, coma
- Hypersomnia
- Akinetic mutism
- Disorientation to time and place
- Antegrade amnesia
- Transcortical motor aphasia.

MAJOR ARTERY STROKES IN POSTERIOR CIRCULATION

Superior Cerebellar Artery Infarcts

Superior cerebellar artery infarcts involves the brainstem territory, ipsilateral Horner's syndrome, contralateral IVth nerve involvement, contralateral loss of pain and temperature, and SCA infarcts with top of Basilar artery involvement.

Clnical Features

- Vomiting
- Dizziness
- Visual field deficits
- Ataxia
- Drowsiness
- Weakness

- Cortical blindness
- Memory loss or confusion

Sometimes coma at initial presentation, tetraplegia and IIIrd nerve palsy may be the feature of occlusion of basilar tip.

Anterior Inferior Cerebellar Artery (AICA) Infarction

General Features

- AICA arises from the basilar artery.
- Supplies inner ear – internal auditory artery.
- There may be brainstem signs at the time of presentation.
- Caudal pons (lateral), middle cerebellar peduncle is the involved territory.
- AICA infarction may be associated with posterior cerebellar artery and superior cerebellar artery infarctions.

Clinical Features

- Vertigo, dizziness, dysarthria.
- LMN VIIth nerve palsy.
- Hearing loss may be sudden (Ipsilateral).
- Horner's syndrome (Ipsilateral).
- Contralateral loss of pain and temperature of the limbs and trunk.
- Coma with tetraplegia may occur in massive ventromedian infarction of the basis pontis.

Posterior Cerebral Artery Infarction

General Features

- Posterior cerebral artery forms the major blood supply of midbrain, thalamus, occipital lobes, and parts of inferior parietal lobe.

- The branches of posterior cerebral artery are: Tubero-thalamic, thalamoperforate, thalamogeniculate, anterior temporal, posterior temporal, calcrine artery and parieto-occipital arteries.
- Clinical features of unilateral PCA are ischemia and infarction.
- TIAS due to atherosclerotic narrowing have an embolic pathogenesis with the source of emboli from the heart, forming majority of infarctions.

Clinical Features

Salient clinical features are:

- Hemiplegia.
- Partial or complete III nerve palsy sensory symptoms.
- Tingling, numbness, burning legs, and slight hemiparesis.
- Ataxia, clumsiness, choreiform movements.
- Visual loss – Contralateral hemianopia, photophobias, hallucinations in the affected field, and complex visual phenomenon.
- Macular sparing (Blood supply is by middle cerebral artery).
- Higher cortical deficits.
- Alexia without Agraphia.
- They can write, speak and spell normally, but cannot read words or name colors.
- Alexia with agraphia, abnormalities reading, writing spelling.
- Amnesia.

Pathogenesis

Pathogenetic mechanisms are:
- Cardiac emboli
- Migraine
- Coagulopathy.

Bilateral PCA Infarction

Clinical Features

- Cortical blindness (Bilateral infarction of striate cortex).
- Denial of blindness.
- Visual cofabulation.
- Normal pupillary reaction to light.
- Amnesia (bilateral infarction of the temporal lobe).

Pathogenesis

- Atherosclerotic plaques.
- Emboli to top of the basilar artery or thrombosis.
- Hypertensive encephalopathy.
- Uremia.
- Eclampsia.

LACUNAR INFARCTIONS

Lacunae are lesions < 1.5 cm in diameter. They are commonly found in the basal ganglia, pons, internal capsule, thalamus and centrum semiovale.

Pathogenesis

They may occur due to the following underlying following pathogenetic mechanisms:
- Atherosclerosis

- Cardiac emboli
- Angiopathies
- Poorly controlled diabetes
- Hypertension
- Lacunes are invariably due to small vessel disease.

Clinical Features

- Dementia: (Thalamus)
- Pure motor hemiplegia
- Cerebellar infarction
- Dysarthria
- Clumsy hand
- Pure sensory stroke (Hemianesthesia, pain, temperature).

STROKE IN YOUNG PATIENTS

General Features

- Can be defined as stroke in individuals less than 40 years in age
- No obvious cause has been found
- Many cases have been reported from India
- Large vessel involvement: ICA, MCA ACA and vertebrobasilar artery.

Pathogenesis

- Diabetes mellitus
- Migraine
- Collagen vascular disease.

In women, the causes are:
- Aneurysm or AVM, with or without hemorrhage.
- Leukemia

- Aplastic anemia
- Oral contraceptive use
- Cerebral thrombosis during pregnancy and puerperium.

Cardiac causes include:

- Mitral valve prolapse
- Atrial fibrillation
- Atrial septal defect
- Patent foramen ovale
- Cardiac tumors.

Other causes of stroke in the young:

- Primary antiphospholipid antibody syndrome
- SLE
- Moyamoya disease.

Moyamoya syndrome: Obstruction of carotid arteries occurs at the siphon. It is defined by angiographic appearance of the collateral circulation, showing hazy appearance on the angiogram, also known as "cigarette smoke" appearance. The following pathological features are observed: Endothelial fibrosis and hyperplasia and absence of any inflammatory change. The following clinical features may be present: Cognitive decline, headache, seizures, etc.

Ischemic stroke due to migraine: This is usually due to small vessel infarction. Ischemic symptoms, referable to retina and occipital cortex may occur Headache can be either occipital / frontal in location.

Cardiac arrhythmias:

- Atrial fibrillation
- Sick sinus syndrome: Changing P wave contour and chaotic atrial activity
- Runs of atrial/nodal tachycardia

- Sinoatrial arrest
- Atrial flutter
- Romanoward syndrome
- Long QT interval (ECG).

Subacute bacterial endocarditis: Staphylococcus aureus and *group D Streptocococcus* are the most common organisms involved, which occur in the setting of calcified valves, prosthetic valves, MVP, rheumatic valves, etc. Clinical features **may include,** intermittent fever, fatigue**, backache, and loss of weight and appetite. Pathological features may include the following:**

- Chronic white matter changes, suggestive of microvasculopathies (Binswanger's disease);
- Occipital lobe and periventricular white matter involvement may be predominant
- Patchy demyelination: Corpus callosum, and cortex are spared
- Penetrating arteries are thickened and hyalinized
- Rarely, amyloid deposits may be present in the vessels of the cortex.

CADASIL (Cerebral Arteriopathy with Subcortical Infarcts and Leukoencephalopathy)

The onset usually occurs in the early 40s. There may be migraine type headaches. The chromosomal locus involved is chromosome 19Q12. There may be dementia, lacunar stroke and/ or pseudobulbar palsy. On MRI imaging, periventricular T2 weighted lesions are prominent. Patchy areas of myelin abnormality may be present.

CEREBRAL HEMORRHAGE

Major causes of cerebral hemorrhage are:

- Hypertension
- Aneurysm, AVM, cavernous hemangioma.

- Medical causes of platelet or clotting factor dysfunction.
- Anticoagulation
- Bleeding into the tumor
- Trauma
- Alcohol.

Hypertensive Hemorrhage

Sites

- Basal ganglia (caudate, putamen, globus pallidus)
- Thalamus
- Cerebellum
- Pons
- Medulla
- Midbrain.

Clinical Features

- Sudden rise of blood pressure is caused by manoeuvers such as heavy lifting, coitus, vomiting, coughing, and straining.
- Majority of the patients are lethargic, stuporose or comatose, but significant proportion are alert.
- Onset: May occur over minutes to hours.
- Headache is present in majority of cases.
- Severe neck-stiffness, positive Kernig's sign, and photophobia suggest rupture of the hemorrhage into the ventricular system.
- Vomiting and nausea occurs at the time of onset due to raised intracranial pressure.
- Usual range of BP is 220-240 mm Hg systolic and 110 – 120 mm Hg diastolic.

- It is important to note that CT scan and MRI are of immense value in management of cerebral hemorrhage. The expansion of the clot occurs over a period of hours and ischemic pneumbra can be delineated and proper therapeutic measures instituted.
- Clinical examination may reveal
  - Enlarged aortic knob.
  - Thickened radial artery.
  - Hypertensive changes in the retina.

Non-hypertensive Causes of Intracranial Hemorrhage

- Vascular malformations
- Aneurysms.

Parenchymal and Subarachonoid Hemorrhage

Clinical Features

- Intense headache, usually of the pounding type
- Vomiting
- Loss of consciousness – Stupor, drowsiness
- Congenital aneurysms usually occur at branch points in the arteries of the circle of Willis.
- Decreased amount of type III collagen
- Defect of arterial media.
- Loss or break in the internal elastic membrane.
- Familial aggregation of congenital aneurysms.
- 7-10% of patients with aneurysmal rupture have first or second degree relatives with an aneurysm.
- If there is familial aggregation, 2-3 members may be affected. The mode of inheritance in these cases is most probably autosomal dominant.

Risk Factors

- Alcohol consumption
- Smoking
- Atherosclerosis
- Hypertension in older men is a particular risk
- 30% may rupture during normal activity.

Symptoms

- Acute onset headache, photophobia, seizures.
- Third nerve palsy.

Chronic Symptoms

- Headache (mass effect)
- Diplopia
- Pyramidal tract dysfunction
- VI, III and IV nerve involvement.
- **Signs of note in ruptured aneurysm:** Subhyloid hemorrhage, neck stiffness, shoulder and back pain.

Specific Clinical Features in an Aneurysm

Posterior Communicating Artery

- Pain behind the eyes
- Partial ptosis
- MRI blood in the suprachiasmatic cisterns.

Anterior Communicating Artery Aneurysm

- Mental status changes
- Agitation
- Amnesia

- Decreased executive function
- MRI: Blood in medial-frontal lobe
- Personality change
- Confabulation.

Internal Carotid Artery Aneurysm

- Pain behind the eyes
- Ptosis
- Pupillary paresis
- Complete IIIrd nerve palsy
- Nasal visual field defect
- Contralateral hemiparesis and hemisensory deficit
- Top of the basilar – PCA bifurcation aneurysm
- Pain in the back of the occiput
- IIIrd nerve palsy
- Visual field defect
- Thalamic sensory deficit
- MRI: Blood in perimesencephalic cisterns.

Medical Complications of Aneurysmal SAH

- 50% may show an abnormal ECG
- 25% may show ST segment or T-wave abnormalities
- Cardiac arrhythmias
  - Tachycardia
  - Bradycardia
  - Atrial fibrillation
- Pulmonary edema, renal dysfunction. Although > 95% of patients show positive changes on CT, lumbar puncture is of definitive diagnostic value.

Miscellaneous Causes of Subarachnoid Hemorrhage

Trauma

This is most commonly due to head injury, which can either result in immediate, or delayed hemorrhage.

Mycotic Aneurysm

- Subacute bacterial endocarditis
- Aspergillosis.

Drug Abuse

- Cocaine abuse
- Heroin abuse
- Amphetamine abuse
- LSD
- Alcohol

The clinical picture of cerebral hemorrhage due to drug abuse is more or less similar with seizures, strokes being common. Hallucinations, mental agitation and false positive serology is commonly seen.

In alcohol abuse: There is acute elevation of blood pressure, concomitant with platelet abnormalities.

Primary Tumors that Hemorrhage

- Glioblastoma multiform
- Pituitary apoplexy
- Metastatic tumors which are hemorrhagic are melanoma, bronchiogenic carcinoma, and choriocarcinoma.

Bleeding Diathesis

- Platelet abnormalities: These abnormalities can cause bleeding from the gums and vaginal bleeding
- Disseminated intravascular coagulation
- Hemophilias
- Thrombolysis related hemorrhage after MI: usually multiple.

VENOUS STROKES

Last trimester of pregnancy and the first month of perineurium, postpartum and due to extreme dehydration.

Clinical Features

- Progressive onset.
- Repeated seizures, vomiting, severe headache, papilledema.
- Sagittal sinus thrombosis presents with focal seizures of the leg.
- Rapid loss of consciousness.
- In cavernous sinus thrombosis: Paresis of III, IV, V, and VI nerves.
- Occlusion of lateral cerebral veins, veins of Galen and straight sinus present with stupor and coma.
- Cortical cerebral venous occlusion presents with focal neurological signs, seizures at the time of presentation, headache, and minimal depression of consciousness.
- *MRI*: Delta sign (what is this sign?) at the confluence of sinuses, bilateral basal, thalamic hemorrhage and small compressed ventricles.

ANTI-IMMUNE DISEASE AND STROKE

Systemic Lupus Erythematosus

Clinical Features

- General neurologic manifestations
- Psychosis
- Sensorimotor neuropathy
- Chorea
- Migraine
- Seizures
- Stroke
- Source of cardiac emboli
- Libman-Sachs endocarditis
- Endocarditis
- Hematologic abnormalities
- Thrombocytopenia
- Arterial microaneurysms
- Platelet thrombi in arteries and capillaries.

Other Autoimmune Causes that Cause Stroke

- Polyarteritis nodosa
- Sarcoid
- Rheumatoid arthritis
- Scleroderma.

Infections that Cause Stroke

Some of the infections which cause stroke include the following:

- Meningococcal infections
- Pneumococcal infections
- *Syphilis:* This could be associated with the brainstem strokes

Associated signs include:

- Argyll Robertson pupil
- Progressive encephalomyelitis
- Peripheral neuropathy
- VDRL in CSF is positive.

Immunologically Compromised Host and Stroke

- Impaired T-lymphocyte or macrophage function.
- Disorders affecting B–lymphocyte function.

These may be due to bacterial, viral or fungal infections.

Amongst the fungal infections, mucormycosis is associated with ethmoid and/ or maxillary sinus infection. It commonly occurs in diabetic ketoacidosis, renal failure, HIV infection. Drug abuse with heroin can result in infections like *Cryptococcus* and *aspergillosis.*

Virus Infections and Stroke

- Immune complex deposition
- Herpes zoster

Delayed brain infarction occurs 6-8 weeks following rash. Carotid occlusion may oocur at the siphon. MCA or ACA occlusion commonly occurs. Rarely posterior communicating artery and vertebrobasilar arteries may also be involved. There may be concomitant encephalitis.

Fungal Infection and Stroke

Cystecercosis

Patterns of infarction:

- MCA
- PCA
- ACA also involves basilar artery.

Clinical features are similar to those oberved in other types of strokes.

12 Epilepsy

The term epilepsy or more correctly epilepsies refers to a group of chronic neurologic conditions characterized by episodes of one or recurrent seizures. Even when there are no overt manifestations of epilepsy that is seizure, neurologic dysfunction may exist for generating seizures. Epileptic seizures are the clinical manifestations (signs and symptoms), resulting due to excessive or hypersynchronous, usually self-limiting, abnormal activity of neurons in the brain. The mechanisms for seizure generation are also present at subcortical level and not purely restricted to cortical level. Epileptic focus has been defined electrophysiologically and now by newer imaging methods as the brain areas that appear to generate the most prominent interictal epileptic form EEG discharges. Thus the epileptic focus may be single, bilateral, independent foci, multiple foci or there may be generalized diffuse epileptic form abnormalities with no focal features.

The area of the brain required to generate even a focal epileptic discharge – seizure is not restricted to any tiny area, but is usually referred to wider area of the brain known as epileptic region. This can only be delineated by clinical features of a seizure such as ictal, or postictal phenomena, electro-encephalography, magnetoencephalography, neuroimaging including atomic force microscopy, spectroscopy, etc. The latter investigations are still being used as research tools, but are very likely to become routine investigative methods in future and would help in exactly delineating the epileptic focus. This would be especially helpful while initiating treatment with medication and surgical methods, e.g. resection of the epileptic region of the brain.

Certain Clinical Terms in a Seizure which Need to be Defined (Figs 12.1A to C)

These include the following:

- Ictal event
- Postictal event
- Aura

Ictal Event

Ictal event refers to the epileptic seizures; postictal event refers to dysfunction after the event is over. Aura may prelude an ictal event by a few seconds or minutes, but also may be manifested hours prior to the ictal event.

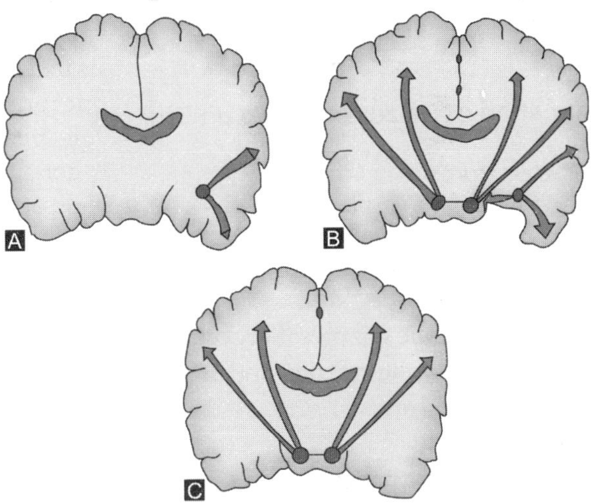

Figs. 12.1A to C: Origins of different types of seizures

The International Classification of Epileptic Seizures

1. *Partial Seizures*

   They are classified on the basis of impairment of consciousness:

   a. Simple partial seizures–No impairment of consciousness.
   b. Complex partial seizures– Impairment of consciousness.
   c. Partial seizures with secondary generalization.

2. *Generalized Seizures*

   These are characterized by involvement of both hemispheres and impaired consciousness levels. They can be classified into the following types:

   - Tonic clonic seizures
   - Absence seizures
   - Myoclonic seizures
   - Atonic seizures
   - Tonic seizures
   - Clonic seizures

Classification of Seizures Based on Etiology

Idiopathic Seizures

- No precipitating central nervous system insult.
- No systemic metabolic dysfunction or history of prior neurologic insult.
- Acute symptomatic seizures that occur one week after acute central nervous system lesion and are not concurrent with:
  - Alcohol withdrawal
  - Febrile episode
  - Metabolic disturbance.

Older Classification International League Against Epilepsy

Classification includes the following, which may be useful for localization of focus of epilepsy:

- Frontal lobe epilepsy
- Temporal lobe epilepsy
- Parietal lobe epilepsy
- Occipital lobe epilepsy.

Some epileptic seizures may be provoked under specific conditions as described below:

- Temperature change
- Photic stimulation
- Simple calculation
- Television, video games
- Chess
- Reading
- Specific tones (Auditory)
- Eating, walking, or singing.

Some seizures may occur under influence of:

- Alcohol – Alcohol withdrawal
- Fever – Febrile seizures
- Drugs
- Eclampsia
- Non-ketotic hyperglycemia.

GENERALIZED SEIZURES

Clinical Features

Prodromal Phase

Prodromal symptoms may include all or some of the following:

- Extreme fatigue, lasting for several days to a week prior to seizure onset

- Mood change
- Increased irritability, headache.

Pretonic/Clonic Phase

Pretonic/clonic phase of a tonic/clonic seizure may comprise of the following:

- Myoclonic jerk
- Brief clonic seizure
- Deviation of head and eyes (frontal and occipital focus).

Tonic Phase

Features of the tonic phase include the following:

- Tonic contraction of axial musculature, resulting in upward eye deviation
- Pupillary dilatation
- Epileptic cry
- Tongue bite
- Jaw contraction
- Cyanosis.

Clonic Phase

Features of the clonic phase include the following:

- Gradually increasing amplitude of the clonic phase
- Incontinence
- Atonia of muscles.

Postictal Phase

Features of the postictal phase include the following:

- Sleep – 30 minutes to one hour
- Confusion on awakening

- Dull pounding headache
- Todd's paralysis
- Increased blood pressure
- Hyperhydrosis
- Temperature is raised
- Postictal psychosis.

Laboratory Features

- CSF cell count: Neutrophils > 100 per mm
- Increased prolactin levels
- Myoglobinuria

Complications of a Seizure

The possible complications of a seizure include the following:

- Fracture dislocation of the shoulder
- Sudden epileptic death
- Severe acidosis.

Etiology

Causes of the generalized tonic clonic seizures include the following:

Genetic Abnormality

The following chromosomal abnormalities may be involved in generalized epilepsy with febrile convulsions:

- Chromosome 5Q 14-15
- Chromosome 8Q 13 – 2
- Chromosome 2

These genes on the involved chromosome principally modulate the expressions of Na^+ channel alpha – subunits.

Clinical features of the tonic clonic seizures due to genetic abnormalities:

- Benign childhood onset
- Simple febrile seizure followed by GTCS
- Complex febrile seizures
- Prolonged duration
- Could be followed by temporal lobe epilepsy in > 25% of patients

Generalized seizures with focal seizures are usually associated with genetic chromosome 19Q 13.1 Na^+ channel mutation.

Metabolic Diseases Causing GTCS

- Hypoglycemia
- Hypocalcemia
- Hypomagnesemia
- Uremia
- Hepatic encephalopathy
- Hyponatremia
- Inappropriate secretion of ADH
- Non-ketotic diabetic coma
- Pulmonary failure
- Drugs.

Hypoglycemia

CSF sugar becomes low as the blood glucose levels falls. The seizures are preceded by hunger, hyperhydrosis, abnormal behavior or low temperature.

Hypocalcemia

General features:

- Fasciculation of muscles
- Chvostek's sign
- Trousseau's sign
- Long QT interval
- Nonspecific T-wave changes

Clinical features:

1. *Hepatic encephalopathy:* Acute onset of impaired consciousness EEG shows slowing with triphasic EEG discharges
2. *Inappropriate ADH secretion follows head trauma, drugs, pulmonary failure* $PCO_2 > 70$ torr; $PO_2 < 80$ torr)
   Serum sodium levels between 120-130 mEq/L
   - Optic fundi: Papilledema
   - Asterexis
   - Fasciculations
   - Generalized seizures.

Infections Causing GTCS

- Bacterial meningitis
- Encephalitis
- Tuberculosis
- Viral encephalomyelitis
- Fungal disease mucormycosis, cysticercosis, etc.
- HIV

Tumors Causing GTCS

- Primary
- Metastatic

Other Causes of GTCS

- Head injury
- Prior history of stroke
- Alcohol withdrawal
- Anticonvulsant withdrawal
- Cortical thrombophlebitis

ABSENCE SEIZURES

Onset of absence seizures occurs between 3-6 years of age. Such seizures rarely persist into adulthood. These seizures last for less than 30 seconds and are not preceded by any aura.

Simple Typical Absence

Features

- Sudden onset of impaired consciousness
- Associated with absence of facial expressions
- Absence of any motor or behavioral manifestations.

Complex Typical Absence

It is accompanied by motor, behavioral and autonomic features. It may be characterized by sudden onset of blank stare, eyeblinks, nystagmus, and rapid arm jerking.

Automatisms

These are acts of semi-purposeful movements and behaviors which the patient cannot recall. These may include movements such as hand rubbing, licking of lips, chewing, picking at clothes, perseverative speech or frank dysarthria.

Autonomic features include pupillary dilatation, hyperhydrosis, salivation, urinary incontinence, etc.

Absence Syndromes

Lennox-Gastaut Syndrome

- Onset: Occurs prior to the age of 5
- Tonic/clonic, or absence seizures
- There also may be myoclonic jerks.
- EEG may show spike and waves less than 3 Hz and abnormal background abnormalities.

Childhood Absence

- Simple or complex
- Genetic predisposition
- Girls are frequently affected
- Frequency of absences: May be greater than 100 in a day
- EEG shows bilateral, symmetrical and synchronous 3 Hz spikes and wave discharges
- 25% of patients with absence seizures may develop GTCS later in life.
- Absences may remit in late life-adulthood.

Absence Status Epilepticus

- Sustained impairment of consciousness
- Confused state of mind
- Facial twiching, eye blinking, automatisms, staring
- EEG shows generalized irregular activity, comprising of approximately 3 cycles/second spike and wave discharges. There may be prolonged bursts of discharges.

- Nocturnal absence status, language and cognitive decline, NREM sleep spike and slow wave.

MYOCLONIC EPILEPSY

Progressive Myoclonic Epilepsy

Causes

- Inborn errors of metabolism
- Genetic disorders
- Lysosomal storage disease
- Lafora's body disease
- Gaucher's disease
- Dawson's encephalitis.

Myoclonic Syndrome

- West syndrome
- Infantile spasms.

Clinical Features

- Retarded psychomotor development
- Hypsarrhythmia on EEG
- Familial myoclonic epilepsy
- Extremity myoclonus
- Cortical tremor familial onset
- Somatosensory evoked giant potentials.

Genetic Abnormality

- Chromosomal involvement at 8Q 24
- Autosomal dominant mode of inheritance
- Adult onset.

MERF (Mitochondrial Encephalomyopathy with Ragged Fibers)

- Short stature
- Diabetes mellitus
- Sensory neural hearing loss
- Proximal limb weakness
- Progressive myoclonic epilepsy.

PARTIAL SEIZURES

- Simple motor partial seizures
- Motor signs and symptoms depend upon the area of the motor cortex activated.

Simple Sensory Partial Seizures and Motor Seizures

Jacksonian March

Thumb initiates clonic movements followed by twitching of the corner of the mouth and the arm. The twitching then spreads to distal leg as in simple motor partial seizures.

Simple partial sensory seizures:
- This type of seizure stimulates same topographical area as in motor seizures.
- Patient complains of spreading tingling numbness.
- According to anatomical locations, the following areas of the brain may be affected:
  - Occipital lobe: Partial sensory seizures may emanate from occipital lobe. Involvement of area 17 is associated with non colored flashes of light, scotomata, and blindness; area 18, and 19 are associated with moving geometric forms which are colored or patterned.

  - If from the occipital lobe there is spread to temporal lobe, then seizure pattern may differ. There may be complex, visual images, microspia, and visual hallucinations.

TEMPORAL LOBE EPILEPSY

Clinical Features

- *Visceral auras*: There may be visceral auras. Aura can be defined as an ictal event occurring before the loss of consciousness. These could be of the following types:
  - *Olfactory auras*: Unpleasant smells such as that of burning rubber may be produced by stimulation of amygdala, olfactory bulbs, uncus, and posterior orbital frontal cortex.
  - *Gustatory auras*: There may be auras related to taste. There may be pleasant or unpleasant taste sensation, suggestive of rotting matter, chemicals, sweat and blood.
  - *Abdominal aura*: **Epigastric rising sensation, subjective fears of having to defecate,** choking throat sensation, hunger, etc.
  - *Cardiac aura*: Heart pacing arrhythmias.
  - *Visual aura*: Blurred vision; perceptual illusion, objects may appear too far or too close, distorted objects.
  - *Auditory auras*: Receptive aphasia, muffled sounds too loud or too soft sounds noise such as clicking, rumbling, etc.
  - *Vascular auras*: Nonspecific dizziness, severe vertigo.
- Postictal bradycardia.
- Patients with seizure disorder in general have a higher incidence of psychiatric disorders in comparison to the

control population. In TLE psychosis, clinical features resembling paranoid schizophrenia have been reported.
- Aggressive behavior may be observed in TLE.
- There may be defects in the memory: Short-term memory loss, and decreased word fluency.

Localizing Features of Importance in TLE

Medial temporal lobe:
- Abnormal smell and taste sensations
- Feeling of impending doom
- Searching head movements: In this condition, the patient may be in a state of trance and yet exhibit foreward and backward head movements.
- Butterflies in the abdomen.

Lateral temporal lobe:
- Episodes from past life
- Detachment
- Rage

Anterior temporal lobe:
- Panic attacks
- Anxiety
- Swearing
- Pupillary dilatation.

Causes

- MTL (Medial temporal lobe) syndrome
- Hippocampal atrophy: Increased T2 signal, disruption of internal structure of hippocampus
- Loss of cells primarily in CA1 CA3

- Other defects
  - Migrational defects
  - Tumors
  - Porencephaly
  - Vascular malformations.

Hippocampal Sclerosis

This the most common type of neuropathological damage seen in individuals with *temporal lobe epilepsy.*

Clinical features of hippocampal sclerosis

- Deficit in verbal comprehension and verbal memory
- Usually follows prolonged febrile convulsions
- Postictal psychosis
- Autonomic auras
- Amygdala sclerosis
- Pathology: Microscopic variant of cortical dysplasia
- May be produced as a result of vascular lesion, hamartoma, or tumors.

Some special features of note include the following:

- In TLE, 50% of women may show sexual and/or hormonal dysfunction
- 20% have amenorrhea, and reduced fertility
- Men with TLE may also suffer from lack of libido.

Laboratory Findings

- Prolactin levels may be raised after TLE seizures.

Parietal Lobe Lesions and Seizures

Clinical Features

- Abnormal tongue sensation – coldness and numbness

- Other phenomena are that the patient feels that a body part is absent or is being moved.
- There may be sense of disorientation in space, vertigo, severe thermal dysthesiae arising from the feet and moving upwards.
- Dominant parietal lobe lesion may cause receptive or conduction aphasia
- Sometimes painful sensations on the limbs as auras may be the presenting feature of parietal lobe seizures.

FEBRILE CONVULSIONS

General Features

- These seizures usually occur in infancy and childhood between the age of 3 months to 5 years in association with fever, but without any evidence of intracranial cause or infection, including meningitis and encephalitis.
- Simple febrile seizures are usually solitary and last for less than three minutes.
- These are usually generalized tonic clonic seizures.

Complex Febrile Seizure

- Multiple seizures
- Seizure duration > 15 minutes
- In 24 hours, there may be more than one seizure
- There may be focal features related to the seizure.

Risk of Epilepsy

- Risk is four times more than that of control population and is more so in complex febrile convulsions.

- If the febrile seizure occurs below 6 months of age, the risk of developing epilepsy is significantly higher at one year
- Family history of epilepsy and febrile seizures.

Status Epilepticus

- Status epilepticus is defined as a series of seizures merging one into the other that do not cease; consequently there is loss of consciousness and continuous electrical activity.
- The time period for it to be defined as status epilepticus is thirty minutes.
- Usually there is loss of consciousness in all major status types.
- Nevertheless, loss of consciousness may not be absolutely necessary to meet the criteria of definition of status epilepticus
- The duration may vary from a few hours to days.

Types

- Generalized status epilepticus
- Absence status epilepticus
- Simple partial status
- Complex partial status

Generalized status epilepticus is to be treated as an emergency. If left untreated, it leads to irreversible neuronal damage and death from both altered cerebral metabolism and secondary injury due to lactic acidosis, hypercarbia or hyperthermia.

Causes of Status Epilepticus

- Poor antiepileptic drug compliance
- Sudden or recent withdrawal of antiepileptic drugs (AEDs)

- Acute illness such as meningoencephalitis, stroke, head injury, metabolic disturbances or alcohol withdrawal.

Outcome depends upon the age of the patient, underlying conditions and duration of status epilepticus before the treatment is instituted. Inadequate treatment of status epilepticus may leave **sequel** of myoclonic jerks which may be difficult to differentiate from true myoclonic epilepsy and thus appropriate AEDS may not be instituted. The longer this state of status epilepticus is allowed to continue, there is further risk of neuronal loss and permanent cerebral damage.

Absence and complex partial status epilepticus (SE) are referred to as non convulsive status epilepticus (SE). The cardinal features are confusional states with occasional myoclonic jerks and automatisms. Absence status is seen in children, while complex status is seen more often in adults. Both forms of status should be considered as emergency. If left untreated, it may lead to permanent cognitive impairment.

Epilepsia Partialis Continua

This is a rare epileptic manifestation with narrow etiological diagnosis.

More often it presents in form of focal twitching of limbs, face or part of the body.

Etiologies include: A structural lesion such as tumor, cortical dysplasia, Rasmussen's encephalitis or inborn error of metabolism.

GENETICS AND EPILEPSY

Genetic epilepsies are those which are directly designated by altered expression of antigens in the chromosomes.

Neonatal beningn familial neonatal convulsions.

Genetics

The defect is in the chromosome 20 Q, which codes for voltage gated K^+ channels.

Clinical features:

- Brief multifocal convulsions.
- First week of life.
- Spontaneous, resolution within six weeks, febrile convulsions may be present.

Juvenile Myoclonic Epilepsy

This may have onset in adolescence or early teenage years.

Genetics

- Autosomal dominant or autosomal recessive mode of inheritance.
- Defect is usually in chromosome 6Q.

Clinical Features

- Early awakening on myoclonus may be present
- Some idiopathic generalized epilepsies may be associated with juvenile myoclonic epilepsies or childhood absence epilepsies, but have different chromosomal defects which may be associated with 8Q chromosome, or 15 Q chromosome.

Other well defined epileptic syndromes having chromosomal defects are described below :

Unverricht's Lundberg disease:

- Involement of chromosome 21Q
- Autosomal dominant mode of inheritance
- Few percent point mutations may occurs.

Clinical features:
- Onset at 6-15 years of age
- Dementia
- Ataxia
- Tremor
- Photosensitivity.

Prader-Willi syndrome:
- Paternally inherited defect in the same region of chromosome 15Q 11-12
- 70% have deletion in chromosome 15Q 11-13
- Non-deletion cases: Both chromosome 15 are from the mother
- Incidence is approximately 1 in every 10,000 live births
- Hypogonadism
- Mental retardation
- Hunger
- Short stature

Tuberous sclerosis:
- Autosomal dominant mode of inheritance with variable expression
- Chromosome 9 link others to chromosome 16
- Tuberous sclerous is a genetic disorder with autosomal dominant pattern of inheritance; two-third of cases occur due to genetic mutations and not due to inheritance. The affected genes may be mapped to the genetic loci TSC1 and TSC2. TSC1 located on the chromosme 9Q34 encodes for the protein hamertin, while TSC2 which encodes for the protein tuberin is located on the chromosome 16p133.

Clinical features:
- Seizures
- Retinal features

MRI:
- Poorly differentiated cortical gyri
- Subpendymal nodules.

Epilepsy syndromes with single gene mutations:
- SCNIB – Sodium channel submit generalized epilepsy with febrile seizures.
- KCNQ2 benign familial neonatal convulsions.

Seizures during Pregnancy

- These can occur in patients with generalized seizures or other types of seizures
- In 24% of women seizures are increased during pregnancy
- These are most frequent at the end of the first trimester and beginning of second trimester

Seizure frequency is dependent upon factors like:
- Seizure type
- Seizure frequency prior to pregnancy
- Intestinal absorption of anticonvulsants
- Hepatic metabolism
- Urinary excretion
- Protein binding
- Hormonal effect

  For instance estrogen increases cortical excitability and progesterone suppresses epileptic discharges.

Differential Diagnosis of Seizure vs Syncope

History about the episode must be elicited from the patient and if bystanders are available, history must also be taken from the bystanders.

Syncope

Syncope usually results from abrupt or gradual reduction of cerebral blood flow. Patients feel lightheaded, faint and may have muscle weakness and gastrointestinal symptoms.

Vasovagal syncope**:** Patient is pale, has bradycardia, and may have cold extremities with sweating. The episode lasts for less than 30 seconds. There is no postictal confusion or amnesia related to the event.

Sphincter disturbances are rare.

Vasomotor syncope:
Following a period of prolonged bed rest, patient feels light headed and may collapse. This may commonly occur after a major illness such as in postcardiac infarction when the patient suddenly rises from supine position. He may collapse without warning and become unconscious for few seconds to minutes. Pallor is the striking feature, pulse may be thready, extremities are cold and clammy and the blood pressure is very low . The patient usually recovers within a few minutes.

***Carotid sinus syncope*: Occurs** due to hypersensitivity of the sinus, tight collar, head turning, etc. Sometimes tonic/clonic seizures may follow syncope.

Cardiac syncope: Cardiac causes includes atrial septal defect tight mitral stenosis, tetralogy of Fallot subaortic stenosis, and cardiac arrhythmias. The following cardiac arrhythmias can result in syncope:

- Artial fibrillation
- Conduction block – Stokes-Adams attack
- Nodal arrhythmias
- Atrial block
- Wolff-Parkinson-White syndrome
- Ventricular arrhythmias.

Other causes of syncope include the following:

- Postural hypotension
- Drugs
- Shy Drager syndrome
- Guillain-Barré syndrome
- Diabetic neuropathy
- Hypoglycemia: This is characterized by stage wise loss of consciousness, hunger, and behavioral change. For further fall of blood sugar, there may be parasympathetic response of salivation, smaller pupils, loss of consciousness and seizures. Pulse may be of normal to low volume and blood pressure may remain unaltered.

Cerebral anoxia causes syncope with clinical features very similar to hypoglycemia, but lethargy, confusion and asterexis are striking features.

Micturition syncope: **Micturition syncope** usually occurs in young men who take in excess of alcohol. This type of syncope usually occurs at initiation of micturition.

Defecation syncope: This type of syncope occurs while straining at stools.

Glossopharyngeal syncope : This usually occurs when a large bolus of food is swallowed. There may be abrupt, but brief loss of consciousness due to overstimulation of posterior pharynx and the cardiodepressor nerves from cranial nerve IX; sometimes in high cervical cord lesions (tumors) and Arnold-Chirari malformation, brief loss of consciousness is associated with severe occipital headache.

SUMMARY

Seizures occur at any time of the day or night. Pallor is absent and is associated with incontinence and tongue biting. Postical confusion is a common feature.

Syncope is classically related to posture have specific triggers and initiating sites. **Pallor** is striking feature of syncope. Urinary incontinence is rare and so is postictal confusion and amnesia. Injury from the ictus is much more common in a **seizure in comparison to the syncope**.

13 Headache

Headache is the most common symptom in medical practice. In general, although eyestrain can result from refractory errors, sinus infection forms significant percentage of headaches. One has to consider migraine tension headache and headache due to raised intracranial tension as separate entities.

MIGRAINE

Site of the Headache

In classical migraine, the site of headache is in the frontotemporal region and is usually unilateral. However, in many cases of migraine, the headache may start in occipital area and migrate to frontotemporal area. Another type of migraine site is that that which mimics sinus disease. In this case, the pain is deep behind the eyes, is usually bilateral and may be aggravated by bright light. The pain may occur in paroxysms. Migraine is more common in females, especially those on oral contraceptive pills or hormonal therapy.

Type of Pain

Throbbing pain is typical feature of migraine headache. It usually starts as mild discomfort and then builds ups to throbbing character before subsiding. Uncommonly at the site of the pain, tenderness can be elicited.

Associated Symptoms

A fortification spectrum is cardinal feature of visual aura. The patient may complain of seeing zigzag lines or complains of loss of vision in one-half of the visual field. They form part of aura. It may show gradual evolution over ten minutes and then clear over the next 20 minutes. All migraine patients do not experience this visual phenomenon. In the majority of patients, there may just be blurring of vision or "watery "eyes or photophobia. During the headache phase, the majority of patients feel nauseated and as the headache subsides there may be vomiting.

Other symptoms include mood changes; the patient may feel irritable or incompetent 24 hours prior to the attack and may find they are making mistakes in their normal day to day activities. On the other hand, sometimes, patients may feel very energetic or "high" and may be surprisingly and unusually productive during the prodomal phase. As a result, when the headache eventually sets in, it is erroneously attributed to over work.

CLASSIFICATION OF MIGRAINE

1. Migraine without aura
2. Migraine with aura
   - Typical aura with migraine headache
   - Typical aura with non-migraine headache
   - Typical aura without headache
   - Familial hemiplegic migraine
   - Sporadic hemiplegic migraine
   - Basilar type migraine.
3. Childhood periodic syndromes that are commonly precursors of migraine

- Cyclical vomiting
- Abdominal migraine
- Beningn paroxysmal vertigo of childhood.

4. Retinal migraine
5. Complications of migraine
   - Chronic migraine
   - Status migrainous
   - Persistent aura without infarction
   - Migrainous infarction
   - Migraine triggered seizures
6. Probable migraine
   - Probable migraine without aura
   - Probable migraine with aura

Migraine without Aura

It is a clinical syndrome characterized by headache features and associated symptoms. There must be at least six attacks fulfilling the following criteria:

- Headache attacks lasting for 4-72 hours.
- Unilateral location
- Pulsating quality
- Moderate or severe pain intensity
- Nausea/vomiting
- Photophobia.

Migraine with Aura

- Typical aura with migraine
- Typical aura without headache
- Basilar type migraine.

Childhood Migraine

- Cyclical vomiting
- Abdominal migraine
- Benign paroxysmal vertigo of childhood.

General Features of Aura

- Most aura symptoms develop over 5-20 minutes and usually last for about 20 minutes on an average.
- Scintillating features with scotoma, visual distortion, microcopies or macroscopsias are more common in children.
- Sensory symptoms include numbness, tingling in face, hand or in hemisensory distribution, dysphasia, in coordination, changes in level of consciousness, etc.

Basilar-type Migraine

- Most often seen in young patients
- Symptoms profile suggest posterior fossa involvement
- Symptoms are bilateral and there may be at least two of the following: dysarthria, vertigo, tinnitus, double vision, ataxia, decreased level of consciousness, etc.

Familial Hemiplegic Migraine

- Autosomal dominant disorder
- Migraine with aura
- Hemiparesis is present.

Childhood Migraine

- Cyclical vomiting syndrome
- Unexplained nausea and vomiting
- The attacks may last for few hours

- There may be intense nausea
- Vomiting is frequent
- There is no abdominal disease
- Common age group includes school children.

Abdominal Migraine

- School children
- Recurrent attacks of abdominal pain
- Anorexia, nausea, and sometimes vomiting
- Pain is poorly localized to the abdominal region
- Physical examination is more or less normal.

Benign Paroxysmal Vertigo

- May affect school children
- Frequent attacks of vertigo
- These may be transient
- Later in life, these children may develop full blown migraine attacks
- Neurological examination is normal
- Audiometric and vestibular function remains normal between attacks
- Electroencephalogram remains normal
- In some cases, multiple episodes of vertigo with vomiting may be present
- Unilateral throbbing headache may be an associated feature.

Retinal Migraine

- Repeated attacks of monocular scotoma or blindness lasting for less than 1 hour

- Age may be less than 40 years
- Normal ophthalmological examination outside attacks
- Retinal infarction may be present.

Menstrual Migraine

- *Pure menstrual migraine*: Migraine without aura usually occurs two days prior to 3rd day of menstruation in at least 2 out of 3 menstrual cycles and at no other time.

Menstrually related migraine: The attacks occur as in pure menstrual migraine, but may also occur at other times of the cycle.

Complication of Migraine

- ***Chronic migraine*** classically occurs in migraine sufferers with migraine headaches lasting for more than 15 days per month for 3 months and no drug overuse.
- ***Status migrainous:*** Headache phase lasts for more than 72 hours despite treatment. All attacks are accompanied by nausea and vomiting. The attack is often debilitating.
- ***Migrainous infarction:*** One or more migrainous aura symptoms are not fully reversible within 7 days and the pathology such as infarction may be confirmed by neuroimaging.
- ***Migrainous epilepsy*** often coexists. Sometimes epileptic seizure is provoked by migraine.

Tension Headache

- Acute type
- Chronic type

- Clinical features are the same, but frequency varies. Stress is the precipitating factor. There may be a tight feeling in suboccipital region, which responds to simple analgesics and stress.
- During the acute attack, there may be severe photophobia. However, drowsiness, nausea, vomiting, incapacitation, etc. are unusual in tension headache.

Headache due to Temporal Arteritis

- **For all headaches** starting after 60 years, temporal arteritis must be considered in the differential diagnosis.
- ESR is elevated.
- There may be immediate response to steroids.
- Associated clinical features are polymyalgia rheumatica, and loss of appetite.
- There may be weight loss, and low-grade pyrexia.
- Headache is generalized and scalp is tender.
- If headache is left untreated, there may be blindness in both eyes.
- Temporal artery biopsy is diagnostic.

Post-traumatic Headache

- There may be tightness in the head and localized tenderness at the site of the trauma. It is usually accompanied by poor concentration, memory disturbance, dizziness, and visual disturbances.

Headache due to Raised Intracranial Tension

- Intense throbbing, pounding headache which is usually generalized.
- Pain may be worsened by movement of the head.
- Headache usually starts building up during the day.
- In later stages the headache may occur throughout the day.
- Patient usually has nausea, vomiting, and intense photophobia.
- Clinical sign of importance is papilledema.

14 Dementia

Causes

Various causes of dementia include the following:

- Alzheimer's disease
- Dementia with Lewy bodies
- Prion disease
- Toxic disorders with dementia
- Neoplasms causing dementia
- Head trauma as a cause of dementia
- Vasculitis and microangiopathic forms of dementia.

Most dementias are now categorized on a molecular, biological, genetic, or neuropathologic basis.

Clinical Features

Basic clinical features of an illness resulting in dementia are:

- *Cognitive impairment:* Cognitive impairment involves multiple domains of cognitive function. The functional representation in dominant and non-dominant cerebral hemispheres is demonstrated in Figure 14.1.
- Deterioration of previously acquired intellectual abilities which interfere with social and occupational function.
- Impairment of memory.
- Disturbances of higher cognitive functions like aphasia, apraxia, and agnosia.

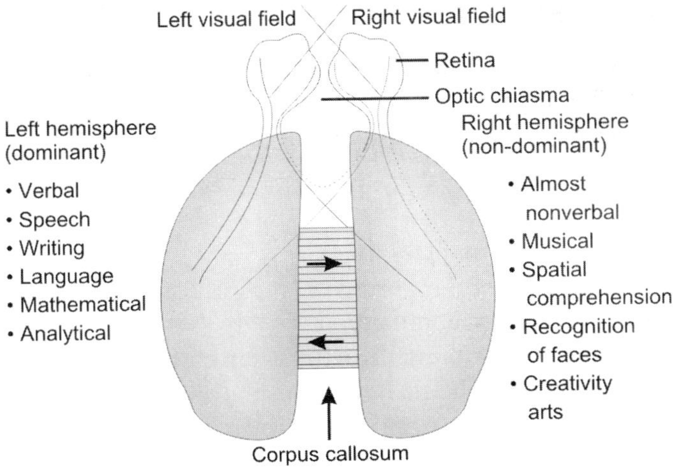

Fig. 14.1: Functional representation in dominant and non-dominant hemispheres

- Personality changes.
- Poor visuospatial abilities.
- Depression, apathy, hallucinations, and delusions.

ALZHEIMER'S DISEASE AND DEMENTIA WITH LEWY BODIES

- Rising prevalence and incidence over the age of 60.
- Genetic factors are commonly present and disease may be familial in 5-10% cases.
- Dementia could be associated with mutations on chromosome 21.
- Early onset dementia: Presinilin I and Presilin II may be the affected genes.
- Late onset AD: Chromosome 19: Apo E4 gene may be involved.

Risk Factors

- Age is the major risk factor.
- Similar incidence worldwide.
- Women are more commonly affected than men.

Pathology

- Extensive neuronal loss.
- Loss of cholinergic neurons of Nucleus Basalis of Meynert and Substantia inominata.
- Intraneuronal neurofibrillary tangles (NFT). Major component of NFT is hyperphosphorylated microtubule associated protein Tau. Earliest evolution of NFT is entorhinal cortex, which progresses to limbic cortex, and finally the last area involved is cortex.
- Amyloid plaques which are extracellular and diffuse.
- Synaptic alterations
- Granulovacuolar degeneration.

Dementia with Lewy Bodies

Clinical Features

- Deficits of frontal subcortical abilities
- Decreased visuospatial skills
- Later memory deficits.
- Associated with parkinsonism – Bradykinesia and tremor
- Poor response to L-dopa.
- Repeated Falls.
- REM sleep disorder, syncope, depression.

Antigenic components of Lewy bodies include presynaptic protein, and alpha synuclein NF proteins. These Lewy bodies occur in temporal lobe. Cortical Lewy bodies are seen in frontal cortex, cingulate gyrus, entorhinal cortex, and amygdala.

Prion disease: In normal healthy brain, prion protein is located on chromosome 20. It is a normal component of neuronal cell membrane. It is transported along axons and accumulates at the neuromuscular junction.

Hereditary form of Prion Disease

This is caused due to the transmission of a mutant prion protein gene, resulting in altered protein production. Mutations of prion protein – different mutations produce different pathologic changes such as, gliosis, amyloidosis, neurofibrillary degeneration, and neuronal loss.

Creutzfeldt-Jakob Disease

- Average rate of infection is 1 case per 1 million people.
- Prolonged incubation period.
- Human transmission has been described to occur from corneal transplant, dural graft, EEG electrodes, etc.
- It is characterized by invariably fatal, rapidly developing dementia with myoclonus.
- Early stages may be associated with gait ataxia, personality changes, dizziness and visual disturbances.
- Late stages may be characterized by aphasia, apraxia, confusion, stupor and myoclonic jerks.

EEG Findings

- Distinctive repetitive sharp waves.
- Periodic complexes.
- 1-2 Hz slow background.

MRI

- Increased diffusion in cortex.
- T2 weighted lesions in the pulvinar.

Pathology

- Cerebral atrophy
- Spongiosis
- Neuronal loss.

HEREDITARY DEMENTIAS

- Alzheimer's disease
  - Presenilin 1 on chromosome 14
  - Presenilin 2 on chromosome 1
  - Trisomy 21
- Creutzfeldt-Jakob disease (chromosome 20)
- Huntington's disease (chromosome 4)
- Parkinson ALS dementia complex of Guam (X-linked)
- Adult onset metachromatic leukodystrophy
- Wilson's disease (chromosome 17)
- Multiple system atrophy
- Olivopontocerebellar atrophy
- Machado-Joseph disease
- Hallervorden-Spatz disease
- Olivopontocerebellar atrophy.

Olivopontocerebellar Atrophy

General Features

- Cerebellar ataxia predominates
- Autonomic dysfunction
- Parkinsonism

Pathology

- Atrophy of cerebellar cortex, vermis, and pons
- Purkinje cell loss
- Neuronal intranuclear inclusions

MRI

- Atrophy of vermis
- Cerebral atrophy

Machado-Joseph Disease

Autosomal dominant disease with involvement of chromosome 14.

Clinical Features

- Varying age of onset.
- Adult onset is most frequent
- Gait ataxia, nystagmus, and external ophthalmoplegia.

Varying Features

- Dementia
- Peripheral neuropathy
- Restless leg syndrome

Amyotrophic lateral sclerosis (Parkinsonism dementia complex of Guam).

General Features

- The disease usually affects Chamoro people of Guam
- Similar disease is also found in the Kii Peninsula of Japan and New Guinea.

Clinical Features

- Motor neuron disease.
- Parkinsonism with severe dementia.

Pathology

- Cerebral atrophy.
- Abundant neurofibrillary tangles.

DEMENTIA DUE TO VASCULAR DISEASE

- More common in males than females.
- Prevalence of dementia is approximately 15% in stroke patients, over 60 years of age.
- About 30% of dementia patients may suffer from vascular disease mixed with Alzheimer's disease.
- In some patients, mental changes are the presenting or only manifestations of stroke.
- Cognitive deficit may be determined by location.

Middle Cerebral Artery

- Acute confusional states with left middle cerebral artery involvement.
- May be associated with infarctions of middle frontal gyrus, middle temporal gyrus, head of caudate nucleus (left).
- Confusional states may last from days to few weeks and occasionally may be permanent.

Anterior Cerebral Artery

- Anterior cerebral artery (ACA) branch occlusions present with dementia. Frontopolar artery, and callosomarginal artery may be involved.

- Clinical signs include mental inertia, apathy, indifference, emotional blunting, etc. This may cause subtle deficits in executive and planning strategies.
- Behavior may be triggered by environmental stimuli.

Posterior Cerebral Artery

- Occipital lobe infarction
- Thalamic nuclear infarction
- Temporal lobe area infarction
- Color naming impaired
- Alexia without agraphia
- Visual distortions and hallucinations
- Bilateral lesions
- Visual agnosia
- Cortical blindness
- Medial temporal lobe infarction
- Severe amnesia
- Usually follows cardiac arrest, severe hypotension
- Anoxia.

Multi-infarct Dementia

- Most common form of vascular dementia
- Patients older than 50
- Men are more frequently involved than women
- Cognitive deficits occur early or late prior to cognitive decline
- There may be gait disturbances and urinary incontinence
- Episodic focal deficits include hemiparesis, ataxia, dysarthria, diplopia, and dysphasia
- Associated medical problems include diabetes, intermittent claudication, myocardial infarction and generalized vascular diseases.

- The lesions may occur in basal ganglia, internal capsule or subcortical white matter.
- The lesions may be bilateral.

MRI Evaluation

- Infarctions in multiple cortical areas
- Lacunar infarction of the basal ganglia, thalamus, internal capsule, and centrum semiovale
- T2 weighted lesions around the ventricles; periventricular white matter lesions prominent on T2 weighted images.
- Ventricular enlargement.
- In lacunar infarction, the degree of dementia accompanies the degree of white matter destruction.
- Numerous microscopic infarcts in the cortex cause cortical granular atrophy.

Binswanger Disease

- Diffuse white matter damage of vascular etiology.

Clinical Features

- Progressive long standing dementia.
- Patients are 50-70 years old.
- Equal affectation of the males and females.
- Hypertensive patients.

Pathology

- Normal brain weight unlike in multi-infarct dementia.
- Atherosclerosis of vessels present.
- Enlargement of third and lateral ventricle, lacunes (lakes) in deep gray matter of pons.
- Minor degrees of cortical infarction, periventricular myelin, pallor.

METABOLIC AND OTHER CAUSES OF DEMENTIA

Renal Failure

- Patients on hemodialysis.
- Slowly progressive course.
- Dysarthria, myoclonus, dysphasia, and seizures.

Uremic Encephalopathy

General Features

- Anemia
- Blood urea > 60 mg/dl.
- Parathyroid hormone may be involved in cognitive changes related to uremia.

Clinical Features

- Cognitive defects in all spheres.
- Memory deficits.

Pathologic Features

- Subdural hemorrhage in 1-30% of patients.
- Generalized neuronal loss.
- Perivascular necrosis and demyelination.
- Areas involved include cerebral cortex, and cerebellum.
- Type 2 astrocytes are prominent.

Liver Failure with Dementia

The severity of dementia caused is directly related to serum ammonia levels.

Clinical Features

- Subcortical dementia
- Falling backwards
- Parkinsonism: Severe dysarthria, choreoathetosis.

Pathology

- Patchy cortical, laminar or pseudolaminar necrosis.
- Diffuse Alzheimer's type 2 astrocytosis.
- Neuronal loss in the cortex, cerebellum and basal ganglia.

Thyroid and Dementia

- Myxedema madness
- Hashimoto's disease
- Apathetic hyperthyroidism.

Clinical Features

- Subcortical dementia
- Lethargy
- Hearing loss
- Apraxia
- Bilateral carpal and tarsal tunnel syndrome
- Sensory motor neuropathy
- Delayed reflexes: Relaxation phase; particularly at ankles.

Laboratory Findings

- Increased CSF proteins and IgG
- Increased interleukin – 6.

Addison's Disease

Due to autoimmune disease.

Clinical Features

- Personality changes
- Apathy
- Cognitive impairment
- Thin muscles (Type II atrophy)
- Depressed reflexes
- Severe fatigue
- Hyperkalemia, low sodium levels (hyponatremia).

Vitamin B_{12} / Folic Acid Deficiency

- Apathy
- Gradual intellectual deterioration
- Optic neuropathy
- Ataxia
- Subacute combined degeneration of the cord.

Folic Acid Deficiency

Cognitive impairment associated with mania.

Chronic Hypoglycemia

- Multiple seizures and coma
- Gradual deterioration of intellectual function, motor neuropathy, involuntary movement, and ataxia.

Neuropathology

- Neuronal loss
- Neocortex layers III-VI are involved
- Purkinje cell loss
- Anterior horn cell loss
- Globus pallidus involvement.

Disorders of Calcium Metabolism

Hypercalcemia

- Cognitive deficits occur when serum calcium levels rise > 13 mg /dL
- Seen in metastatic diseases, hyperthyroidism and hyperparathyroidism.

Clinical Features

- Lethargy
- Stupor
- Impaired cognitive function
- Absent reflexes
- Profound lethargy
- Fasciculating tongue
- Hyperactive reflexes
- Proximal muscle weakness
- Cramps and aches.

Hypocalcemia

Etiology

Hypocalcemia is seen in:
- Uremia
- Vitamin D deficiency
- Pancreatitis.

Clinical Features

- Cognitive impairment
- Neuromuscular irritability

- Chvostek's sign
- Trousseau's sign
- Asterixis
- Seizures
- Basal ganglia calcification.

Cushing's Syndrome

Etiology

- Iatrogenic steroid administration
- Adrenal tumors.

Clinical Features

- Behavioral changes
- Mania, depression
- Psychosis
- Dementia – Subcortical type
- Pseudotumor cerebri
- Proximal myopathy.

DEMENTIA IN ASSOCIATION WITH TOXIC DISORDERS

Aluminum

As implicated in Alzheimer's disease and dialysis dementia.

Alcohol

- Wernicke's-Korsakoff's syndrome
- Alcohol abuse
- Starvation diets
- AIDS

Clinical Features

- Ophthalmoplegia
- Ataxia
- Nystagmus
- Encephalopathy
- Amnesic state
- Normal intelligence and learned memory

Lesions Seen in

- Mamillary bodies
- Periventricular III and IV ventricles.
- In chronic cases Fe^{++} deposition may be seen in mamillary bodies.
- Neuropathological changes seen in cortex white matter, cerebellum and brainstem.

Marchiafava-Bignami Disease

- Usually observed in alcoholics – Male
- First described in male red wine drinkers, may also be seen in non-alcoholics.

Clinical Features

- Seizures
- Disorders of consciousness
- Death
- Progressive dementia
- Interhemispheric disconnection syndrome
- Necrotizing cystic lesions seen in corpus callosum, optic chiasma, centrum ovale and middle cerebellar peduncles
- Axons are usually spared
- MRI shows diffuse swelling of the corpus callosum.

Central Pontine Myelinolysis

- Seen in Wernicke's-Korsakoff's psychosis
- Also seen in patients with severe burns hyponatremia, immunosuppressed states, anorexia, etc.

Clinical Features

- Young or middle aged adults are usually affected
- Flaccid tetraplegia
- Locked-in syndrome
- Facial and pharyngeal paralysis.

Pathology

Lesions extend from the midbrain through the upper 2/3 of the pons principally at the level of VIth nerve nucleus.

Manganese

Dementia can result due to the accumulation of manganese in globus pallidus and substantia nigra.

Clinical Features

- Rigidity
- Akinesia
- Depression
- Poor memory
- Insomnia
- Loss of postural reflexes
- Tremors may be present
- In the late stages, akinetic rigid states, and dystonia may be present.

Pathology

Degeneration of caudate nucleus and putamen.

MRI Evaluation

Increased signal on T2 weighted images of striatum, globus pallidus, and substantia nigra.

Mercury

- Dental amalgam
- Manufacture of scientific instruments.

Clinical Features

- Psychological disturbance with burst of anger
- Intention tremor.

TUMORS CAUSING DEMENTIA

- These tumors can be both benign and malignant
- They may be located in midline.

Colloid Cyst

Obstructional hydrocephalus

Pinealoma

- Clinical features include
- Aqueduct stenosis
- Hearing loss
- Vertical gaze palsy

Pituitary Tumors

These can produce the following defects:
- Chiasmal defects
- Hydrocephalus
- Dementia

Thalamic Tumor

These can produce the following defects:
- Aphasia
- Fluctuating level of consciousness
- **Frontal lobe tumors**
- **Meningioma**
- **Subfrontal tumors**
- Seizures
- Personality and behavioral changes
- Poor memory
- Deficit in attention, executive function and planning.

Lymphoma

- Primarily seen in AIDS patients
- Can produce cognitive decline and frontal lobe syndrome.

Glioblastoma Multiform

- Seizures
- Frontal lobe syndrome.

Paraneoplastic Syndrome

Could be seen in association with the following tumors:
- Small cell carcinoma lung
- Cancer breast

- Cancer ovary
- Cancer GI tract
- Cancer prostate.

Clinical Features

- Memory impairment
- Personality and behavioral changes
- Seizures.

Pathology

- Neuronal loss at the hippocampus and Cingulate gyrus.

HIV AND DEMENTIA

- Microglia and cellular reservoirs of virus.

Clinical Features

- Forgetfulness
- Poor concentration
- Ataxia
- Paraparesis
- CSF protein elevated > 50 mg%
- Lymphocytes are increased.

MRI

- Atrophy of gray and white matter.
- Basal ganglia atrophy.

Associated Pathologies

- Lymphoma
- Progressive multifocal leukoencephalopathy

- Tuberculosis
- Syphilis
- Other viral infections.
- Subacute sclerosing panencephalitis **seen in children with cognitive decline – deterioration in school performance.**
- Apraxia
- Myoclonus.

Pathology

- Cowdry A bodies
- Large intranuclear inclusions.

Laboratory

- Slightly raised protein.
- Few lymphocytes.
- **Multifocal leucoencephalopathy occurs in conditions of immunocompromised disease states:**
  - HIV
  - Renal failure
  - Malignancy
  - Liver disease.

Clinical Features

- Ataxia
- Parietal lobe sensory loss
- Cognitive impairment.

Pathology

- Large multinucleated oligodendrocytes
- Intranuclear inclusions
- Foci of demyelination

Neurosyphilis

- May occur 20 years after the infection
- Memory loss
- Apathy
- Apraxia
- Dysphasia
- Seizures
- Trombone tongue tremor
- Argyll Robertson pupil
- Brainstem strokes.

CSF

- Elevated IgG
- IgM raised in acute infection
- Few cells
- Slight increase in proteins.

Cysticercosis

Infection caused by the larval stage of the pig tapeworm, *taenia solium*.

Clinical Features

- Seizures
- Raised intracranial pressure.
- Hydrocephalus
- Chronic dementia

Pathology

Cysts are found in—
- Cortex
- Ventricles

- Cerebellum
- Meninges
- White matter.

LYSOSOMAL DISORDERS WITH DEMENTIA

GM1 gangliosidosis (type 3)

- Defect involves the chromosome 3
- Defective in protective protein
- Onset may be in the first decade of life.

Clinical Features

- Dementia
- Spasticity
- Dystonia
- Ataxia.

Pathology

- Storage of gangliosides in the cerebral cortex; it is PAS positive.
- Atrophy of caudate, Putamen and Globus pallidus.

Other: Gangliosidosis

- Tay-Sachs disease
- Classical sign: Cherry red spot in the retina
- Seizures
- Mental retardation
- Exaggerated startle response

Niemann-Pick Disease

This disease results due to the deficiency of the enzyme sphingomyelinase.

Clinical Features

- Dementia
- Spasticity
- Seizures.

Metachromatic Leukodystrophy

General Features

- Autosomal recessive mode of inheritance
- Defect in Chromosome 22
- Deficit of aryl sulfatase A

Clinical Features

- Age of onset: 20-50 years
- Impaired concentration
- Memory dysfunction
- Schizophrenia
- Emotional liability.

Pathology

- Loss of myelin throughout the brain
- Deposition of sulfatide in basal ganglia, spinal cord and brainstem nuclei.

Peripheral Nerves

- Loss of myelinated fibers.
- Deposition of sulfatides in macrophages and Schawann cells.

DEMENTIA RESULTING FROM HEAD TRAUMA

Outcome of Blunt head trauma depends on the following two important factors:

1. Duration of coma
2. Resolution of post-traumatic amnesia

Clinical Features

- Subcortical dementia
- Ataxia
- Parkinsonism
- Pyramidal tract dysfunction
- Pseudobulbar palsy
- Dysarthria
- Emotional liability.

Neuropathology

- Diffuse brain damage
- Diffuse axonal injury
- Ischemic brain damage
- Brain swelling with increased intracranial pressure
- Diffuse axonal injury is an important neuropathological feature, which may manifest as focal lesion of the corpus callosum.
- There may be focal lesions in the quadrants of the rostral brainstem.

Dementia Following Repeated Head Trauma

This type of dementia can commonly occur in:

- Boxers
- Football players
- Soccer players

Subcortical Dementia

Clinical Features

- Dysphasia
- Dyspraxia
- Ataxia
- Parkinsonian features
- Pseudobulbar palsy.

Pathology

- Loss of Purkinje cells
- Cortical neuronal loss
- Occipital, temporal, frontal and parietal injury.

MRI Evaluation

- Global atrophy
- Lesions of corpus callosum
- Ventricular dilatation.

DEMENTIA DUE TO DISORDERS OF BLOOD VESSELS

These could include the following disorders:

- Polyarteritis nodosa
- Primary granulomatous angitis
- Giant cell arteritis
- Thrombotic thrombocytopenic purpura
- Systemic lupus erythematous (SLE)

Considering the above mentioned conditions, the clinical features mainly result from damage to the following structures:

- Cranial nerves
- Peripheral nerves

- Spinal cord
- Large or small vessels.

Clinical Features

- Stroke
- CNS involvement may be seen in 20-40% of patients.
- There may be an involvement of large intra- and extra-cranial vessels
- There may be multifocal deficits
- Dementia
- Global encephalopathy
- Seizures
- Large vessel stroke
- Stupor and coma.

Pathology

- Necrotizing vasculitis of small and medium sized muscular arteries
- Segmental lesions
- Polymorphonuclear and mononuclear cell infiltration of blood vessels.

Systemic Lupus Erythematosus (SLE)

Clinical Features

- Large and small cerebral infarcts lead to multi-infarct dementia.
- Presence of lupus anticoagulant anticardiolipin antibodies
- Thrombosis of large and medium sized cerebral vessels.

Laboratory Tests

- False positive syphilis serology
- Prolonged Partial Thromboplastin Time (PTT).

Pathology: Vasculitis

CSF findings: *Increased protein, lymphocytes and IgG levels*

Imaging: MRI shows defects such as atrophy, infarcts.

Primary Granulomatous Angiitis

Arterioles are principally involved; occasionally large intracranial vessels may also be involved.

Clinical Features

- Cognitive decline
- Seizures
- Headache
- Impaired consciousness.

Laboratory

- Segmental narrowing of tertiary blood vessels.

Giant Cell Arteritis

- The most commonly involved vessels are the carotid artery, vertebral artery, and arch of the aorta
- Extracranial blood vessels may be also involved
- There may be brainstem and cerebellar involvement.

Clinical Features

- Severe headache
- Blindness

- Vascular dementia
- Thrombotic thrombocytopenic purpura
- There may be acute confusional state
- Psychosis
- Seizures
- Renal failure
- Vascular dementia
- Purpuric skin lesions
- Age > 60 years
- Sedimentation rate may vary between 80-120 mm.

Pathology

- Granular atrophy of the cerebral cortex
- Organized thrombi.

15 The Brainstem

The anatomy of brainstem is quite complicated. The ventral aspect of the brainstem is shown in the Figure 15.1. It includes medulla oblongata, pons and midbrain. It is stalk-like in shape and connects spinal cord with forebrain.

The brainstem serves four major functions:

1. Various ascending and descending tracts that connect the spinal cord to the different parts of the forebrain pass through the brainstem.

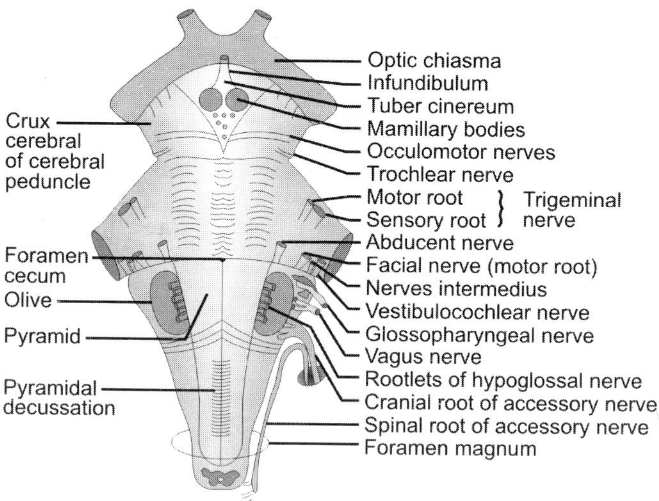

Fig. 15.1: Ventral aspect of the brainstem

2. Has important autonomic reflex centers associated with the control of respiration and cardiovascular system.
3. It is associated with consciousness.
4. It contains important nuclei of (3rd to 12th) cranial nerves.

MEDULLA OBLONGATA

It measures about 3 cm in length, 2 cm in breadth and 1.2 cm in thickness.

It contains vital structures such as:

- Cardiac center
- Vasomotor center
- Respiratory center

It also provides attachment to last four cranial nerves.

The medulla also contains central canal which widens in the upper part and moves dorsally to form the lower part of the fourth ventricle. It is divided symmetrically into right and left halves by anterior median fissure and posterior median sulcus. Anterior median fissure ends into a small triangular depression called foramen cecum. Posterior median fissure above diverges to form the lower part of the floor of the 4th ventricle.

The ventral aspect of the medulla presents the following structures:

1. Pyramids
2. Olives
3. Rootlets of the hypoglossal nerve
4. Inferior cerebellar peduncles.
5. Rootlets of the 9th, 10th, and 11th cranial nerves.

Pyramids are rounded elevations, one present on either side of anterior median fissure and produced by corticospinal (pyramidal) fibers. 75% of fibers cross to the opposite side

(Pyramidal decussation) in the lower part of the medulla and then descend as lateral corticospinal tract in the lateral white column of the spinal cord. 20% of fibers which are uncrossed run downwards as anterior corticospinal tract in the anterior white column of the spinal cord, while the remaining 50% run downwards along with uncrossed fibers in the lateral white column of the spinal cord.

Features of the Posterior (dorsal) Aspect of Medulla

It is demarcated into lower closed and upper open parts. The closed part contains fasciculus gracilis, fasciculus cuneatus and inferior cerebellar peduncle. The upper parts of cunneati form tubercles called respectively as gracile and cunneati tubercles.

The open part forms lower part of the floor of the fourth ventricle which contains median sulcus, hypoglossal and vagal triangles, vestibular areas, and area postrema.

Blood Supply of the Medulla

1. Two vertebral arteries
2. Anterior and posterior spinal arteries.
3. Anterior and posterior inferior cerebellar arteries
4. Basilar artery.

PONS

It lies between midbrain and medulla in the posterior cranial fossa anterior to the cerebellum. It is continuous on either side as middle cerebellar peduncle forming a bridge between two cerebellar peduncles.

Blood Supply

Numerous branches from the basilar artery and anterior inferior cerebellar artery.

Structural Format

- Structurally, the pons consists of gray and white matter containing nuclei and fiber tracts.
- Important attachment of the ventral surface of the pons is trigeminal nerve with its two rootlets: motor and sensory.
- Basilar part comprises of longitudinal bundles of fibers:
  - The corticopontine fibers
  - The corticospinal fibers
- Pontine nuclei are scattered among longitudinal and transverse fibers.
- The pontine nuclei form an important part of the cortico – pontocerebellar pathway which connects the cerebral cortex of one side to the cerebellar hemisphere.
- The tegmental part contains the nuclei of trigeminal, abducens, facial and vestibulocochlear nerves.
- The median leminicus (white matter) is situated in the most anterior part of the tegmentum. It contains fibers for nucleus cuneatus and nucleus gracilis.

MIDBRAIN

Midbrain is about 2.5 cm long and 2.5 cm wide. It connects hindbrain with the forebrain. Its cavity or the cerebral aqueduct connects the third ventricle with fourth ventricle.

It like other parts of brainstem consists of gray and white matter.

The occulomotor nucleus lies in the ventromedial part and is bounded laterally by median longitudinal fasciculus

(Edinger-Westphal nucleus) which supplies ciliary muscles and sphincter pupillae.

Pretectal nucleus is an important part of neurons and lies deep to the superolateral part of the superior colliculus. Its afferents are from the lateral root of the optic tract and gives efferents to the Edinger-Westphal nucleus.

It is an important pathway for pupillary light reflex and consensual light reflex. An important condition arising out of lesion of the pretectal nucleus is Argyll Robertson pupil in which light reflex is lost but accommodation reflex remains intact.

Red Nucleus

It is a cigar shaped mass of gray matter and is situated dorsomedial to the substantia nigra.

Afferent Fibers

Afferents cerebellorubral fibers pass through contralateral dentate nucleus of the cerebellum through superior cerebellar peduncle.

Other connections include:
- Corticorubral fibers from ipsilateral motor area.
- Pallidorubral fibers from the globus pallidus.
- Fibers form the hypothalamus and substantia nigra.
- Fibers from tectum and subthalamic nucleus.

Efferent Fibers

- Rubrospinal tract
- Rubrobulbar tract
- Rubroreticular tracts

- Fibers from rubrospinal tracts end in the motor nuclei of 5th and 7th cranial nerves and also in the nuclei of 3rd and 4th and 6th cranial nerves.

White Matter

Important composition of the white matter is Medial Longitudanal Fasciculus (MLF) which lies ventrolateral to the occulomotor nucleus. It is a heavily myelinated composite tract found in paramedian plane of the brainstem. It consists of fibers arising mainly from vestibular nuclei. The chief function of MLF is to coordinate the movements of eyes, head and neck in response to stimulation of the vestibulocochlear nerve.

Reticular Formation

It comprises of diffusely aggregated network of neurons throughout the lateral parts of medulla, pons and midbrain. It is an ill defined space between cranial nerve nuclei and olives within ascending and descending traces of the brainstem and receives sensory input from the spinal cord, cerebellum and cranial nerve nuclei and sends efferent fibers to these structures. The location of reticular formation in the brainstem is shown in Figure 15.2.

Blood Supply

- Basilar artery through its posterior cerebral and superior cerebellar arteries.
- Branches of posterior communicating and anterior choroidal arteries.

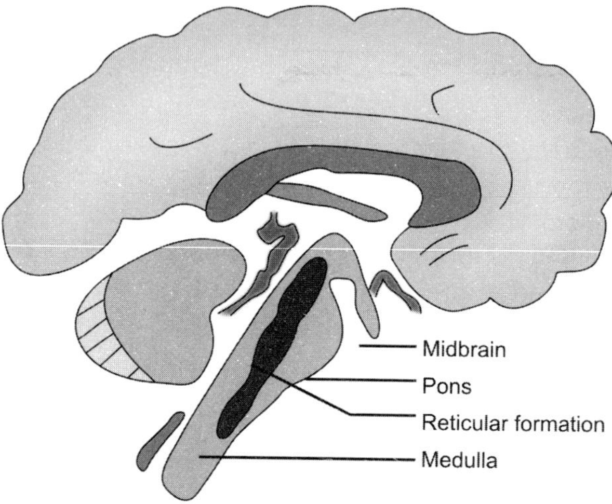

Fig. 15.2: Brainstem: Showing the location of reticular formation

Clinical Aspects of Brainstem Disease

The symptomatology of brainstem disease is important and is primarily acute. Common symptoms include diplopia, dysarthria, vertigo, nausea and vomiting.

Vascular Syndromes

- Midbrain vascular lesions arise from occlusion or embolism of penetrating branches derived from vertebral, and basilar arteries.
- It influences stretch reflexes and muscle tone
- Importantly it has modulatory influence on cardiovascular activities, respiration, arousal, behavior and pain.
- Occlusion of anterior spinal arteries, with consequent blockage of penetrating branches may lead to extensive unilateral or even bilateral infarction at central medullary level.

Dorsolateral Infarction

- It will cause Horner's syndrome on the same side with total loss of sensation on the opposite side.
- Associated features are cerebellar deficit on the same side if superior cerebellar peduncle is damaged. With it if occulomotor nucleus is damaged, there will be combination of 3rd nerve lesion and cerebellar signs with Horner's syndrome on the same side and sensory deficit to all sensations on the opposite side.

Paramedian Infarction

- Damage to the nucleus itself or nerve fascicle
- Damage to the Red nucleus interrupts the dentatorubro-thalamic tract from the opposite cerebellar hemisphere.
- It is characterized by following signs and symptoms and is designated as *Benedikt's syndrome.*
  - Ipsilateral squint and ptosis
  - Contralateral loss of pain and temperature sensation
  - Contralateral loss of tactile, muscle, joint and vibration sense
  - Contralateral tremors and involuntary movements in the limbs.

Perinaud's Syndrome

General features:

- Lesion in the superior colliculi
- Loss of upward gaze
- The syndrome results due to thrombosis of superior cerebellar artery.

Clinical features:
- Downward gaze palsy
- Bilateral upper midbrain infarction
- Combined up and downward gaze palsies
- Bilateral or unilateral midbrain infarction.

There may be the following associated clinical signs:
- Coma and hypersomnia
- Akinetic mutism
- Disorientation of time and place
- Antegrade amnesia
- Delayed athetoid or clonic movements.

Basal Infarction

Third nerve fascicle itself is damaged resulting in complete 3rd nerve palsy. Damage to cerebral peduncle will result in hemiplegia of opposite limbs including face.

Pontine Vascular Lesions

Dorsolateral Infarction

Horner's syndrome on the side of the lesion will be found in nearly all cases coupled with loss of pain and temperature in sensation in the limbs on the opposite side of the body.

Depending upon the level of the lesion in the pons, the associated clinical signs involving sensations and lesions of other cranial nerves are seen.

- **Above midpontine level,** facial sensations are spared and the sensations of touch and propioception remain intact.
- **Below midpontine level,** there occurs loss of sensation over the face on the same side as the lesion due to damage to afferent and efferent fibers of the fifth nerve.

- **At midpontine level**, there will be loss of conjugate lateral gaze towards the side of the lesion.
- At lower pontine level, vestibular and cochlear nuclei are likely to be damaged causing vestibular symptoms, nystagmus and deafness. Associated features include loss of pain and temperature sensation over the face on the side of the lesion.

Paramedian Infarction

Characteristically, lesion is at the level of the **sixth nerve nucleus.** Sixth nerve palsy is combined with a conjugate gaze palsy and facial nerve paresis. Due to the affectation of **median longitudinal fasciculus,** there will be loss of touch and propioception on the opposite side.

Basal Infarction

- Fascicles of sixth and seventh nerves are damaged
- Presence of ipsilateral squint
- Ipsilateral facial palsy
- Contralateral hemiplegia due to involvement of corticospinal tract.

This is designated as Millard-Gubler syndrome.

Medullary Vascular Lesions

Dorsolateral Infarction

This results due to thrombosis of posterior inferior cerebellar artery. This is designated as Wallenberg syndrome. Posterior inferior cerebellar artery supplies dorsolateral part of the medulla and is a branch of the vertebral artery. It also supplies inferior part of the cerebellum. Contralateral loss of pain and temperature sensation in the trunk and limbs occur due to involvement of spinothalamic tract.

There is ipsilateral loss of pain and temperature sensation over the face due to involvement of the spinal nucleus and tract of the trigeminal nerve.

In the upper brainstem, the vascular lesions produce unilateral damage which does not transgress the midline.

Central medullary lesions produces 12th nerve palsy on one side with hemplegia and sensory loss to touch and joint position sensations on the opposite side.

Locked-in syndrome is manifested when there is bilateral infarction. The patient is fully conscious, quadriplegic, becomes mute and is unable to communicate. There is bilateral 12th nerve lesion and loss of touch and position sense in the limbs. Face is spared and if decussating fibers of trigeminal nerve are damaged, there may be bilateral loss of sensation over the face.

Transient Ischemic Episodes

- The symptoms may include vertigo, dysarthria and tingling around the mouth indicating ischemia.
- Central medullary dysfunction.
- If the ischemia is at the pontine level, there may be unilateral numbness, diplopia and hearing abnormalities.
- Majority of these transient ischemic episodes in the posterior circulation are due to emboli traversing vertebral and basilar arteries.
- Sometimes, isolated ischemia in the blood supply region of the posterior cerebral artery occurs, which can give rise to

unilateral weakness of limbs or complete blindness or transient hemianopia associated with vertigo and sudden loss of consciousness.

Brainstem Hemorrhage

Pontine Hemorrhage

- In **acute state of pontine hemorrhage, the** patient complains of severe headache and becomes unconscious, develops periodic breathing, pinpoint pupils, and loss of 'Doll's eye movement' and spastic tetraplegia.
- The spasticity seen in brainstem hemorrhage is usually immediate and is followed by decerebrate posturing.
- Cerebellar hemorrhage is important to recognize. In these cases, the onset is acute with sudden occipital headache, vomiting, ataxia, loss of consciousness, gaze palsies, bilateral pyramidal signs and periodic breathing.
- It may mimic primary **subarachanoid hemorrhage**. Age is the differentiating point as aneurysm in the posterior fossa usually occurs in younger age group as opposed to **cerebellar hemorrhage** due to atherosclerosis which is seen in older age group.
- The importance of delineating various vascular syndromes of the brainstem lies in intelligently applying newer imaging modalities to select patients for appropriate surgical procedures such as stenting in the vertebrobasilar artery syndromes and evacuation of the clot in **cerebellar hematoma**.

Multiple Sclerosis and Brainstem

The hallmark of multiple sclerosis plaque affecting the brainstem are the cardinal signs of cerebellar and pyramidal affectation giving rise to dysarthria, ataxia, brisk reflexes and spasticity with extensor plantars.

Isolated cranial nerve involvement many a times may herald the first attack of multiple sclerosis. For instance, facial numbness due to involvement of fifth nerve in the brainstem with quick recovery over weeks followed by painful trigeminal neuralgia again with recovery may be the 1st sign of brainstem demyelinating plaque.

The medial longitudinal bundle when affected by demyelination produces signs which are characteristic of multiple sclerosis in the presentation of internuclear ophthalmoplegia.

Isolated 6th nerve lesion of lower motor neuron type is the only cranial nerve lesion occurring in multiple sclerosis. Various symptoms may point towards vestibular affectation in the brainstem such as nystagmus, which may be rotatory type or on lateral gaze may be manifested with an early symptom of true vertigo.

Again, newer imaging modalities such as MRI scan and positron emission help in the diagnosis. Tomography does help in localizing the lesions of the brainstem. Sometimes in very early stages, associated white matter lesions in the cerebral hemisphere give a clearer picture of multiple sclerosis with the use of newer imaging modalities.

Tumors of the Brainstem

Gliomas of the pons are seen in children. The presentation may be acute and mimic multiple sclerosis with isolated sixth nerve and seventh nerve palsies. Minimal motor signs and extensor plantars and absent sensory deficit may further complicate the clinical picture.

Again, age is an important differentiating feature, with multiple sclerosis being exceedingly rare below the age of 10 years.

Other tumors such as neurofibroma involving cerebellar peduncles directly infiltrate the brainstem. Similarly astrocytomas of cystic type do mechanically distort the brainstem and give rise to brainstem signs. Ependymomas of the 4th ventricle block cerebrospinal fluid pathway and give rise to rapid hydrocephalus and thus present as nausea, vomiting and papilldema.

Posterior Fossa Tumors

Primary tumors are rare in childhood. Metastatic lesions in the brainstem are much common.

Tumors of the 8th nerve or the acoustic nerve give rise to the signs of brainstem affectation by causing distortion of the brainstem.

Chordomas, cholestatomas and menigiomas are primary tumors of the brainstem usually seen in adults producing signs of brainstem dysfunction along with cranial nerve palsies, cerebellar signs and pyramidal deficit.

Vascular malformation such as angioma, arteriovenous malformation of the basilar, vertebral and posterior cerebral arteries may compress the brainstem at various levels giving rise to the brainstem signs. Similarly due to atherosclerosis, ectasia of the basilar artery may form a tortuosity and saccular aneurysm which can act as space occupying lesion.

It is the development of better imaging systems which has helped in arriving at the correct diagnosis of these space occupying lesions and differentiating them from **Multiple Sclerosis.**

Infections giving rise to Brainstem Signs

These may be primary and could be viral, bacterial, or fungal in orgin.

- *Viral infections:* Amongst the viral infections, the commonest ones are *Herpes simplex* encephalitis, and *Herpes zoster* affecting Vth Nerve.
- *Bacterial infections:* Though primary granulomas due to syphilis are rarely seen, meningovascular syphilis with arteritis of the basilar and vertebral arteries can give rise to a clinical picture simulating brainstem stroke.
- Tubercular arteritis and Moya Moya Disease can involve posterior circulation and thereby produce a picture suggestive of brainstem disease in acute stages.
- *Fungal infections:* Fungal granulomas, cryptococcosis, and mucormycosis may produce a slow growing tumor like presentation.

One condition which needs to be mentioned is brainstem encephalitis, which presents with disturbed consciousness, autonomic signs, tetraplegia with sensory deficit affecting pain, temperature and propioceptive sensation and pyramidal signs in the form of extensor plantars.

Reflexes may be depressed, absent or brisk. The picture mimics ascending Guillain-Barré like syndrome, and **chronic inflammatory demyelinating neuropathy.**

Newer imaging techniques combined with electromyography, nerve conduction velocities and somato sensory evoked potentials may be useful to pinpoint the exact pathology. The site of the lesion may be at any level in the brainstem. Pontomedullary junction or the midbrain.

One of the conditions commonly seen in clinical practice is **migraine**. A separate clinical variety of migraine seen in young women was described as **Basilar Artery Migraine** and subsequently named as **Bickerstaff's Migraine** wherein predominantly symptoms are referred to posterior circulation.

Brainstem Dysfunction as a Result of Metabolic/Toxic Causes

Toxic effects of alcohol can give rise to brainstem signs in the form of isolated VIth nerve palsy, and internuclear ophthlamoplegia. Trasient pyramidal deficit and **Wernicke's encephalopathy** occurs in chronic alcoholics and in addition to diffuse disturbance of cerebral function– manifested by confusion, confabulation, and retrograde amnesia. There is usually manifestation of brainstem dysfunction which may be in the form of gaze palsies, respiratory depression, autonomic disturbance, pupillary abnormalities, nystagmus and pyramidal signs. These signs are reversible, provided the patient receives **thiamine** intravenously.

Another condition which gives rise to brainstem dysfunction and pathological changes in the pons is central pontine myelinolysis, which can be clearly seen on MRI imaging. It is rare but lethal condition resulting from severe electrolyte disturbance, hypokalemia complicating burns, sepsis, adrenal failure, hepatic disease, etc.

Index

A

H

I

P

T